**Medicaid Decisions:
A Systematic Analysis
of the Cost Problem**

Medicaid Decisions:

A Systematic Analysis of the Cost Problem

Stephen M. Davidson, Ph.D.
The University of Chicago

Ballinger Publishing Company • Cambridge, Mass.
A Subsidiary of Harper & Row, Publishers, Inc.

International Standard Book Number: 0-88410-142-8

Library of Congress Catalog Card Number: 80-10998

Printed in the United States of America

Library of Congress Cataloging in Publication Data
Davidson, Stephen M.
Medicaid decisions.

Bibliography: p. 201
Includes index.
1. Medicaid—Finance. I. Title.
HD7102.U4D278   338.4'3362104252'0973   80-10998
ISBN 0-88410-142-8

For Harriet

Contents

List of Figures

List of Tables

Foreword

It is a pleasure and an honor to be asked to write the Foreword to this book. Stephen Davidson was a student in my seminar on Contemporary Problems and Issues a number of years ago, and this book is an outgrowth of a major research project he prepared on Medicaid for that seminar. Seldom does a professor have the privilege of seeing a seminar project blossom into a full-scale book. My relationship with Davidson has continued to this day both as a friend and colleague. As the latter, I have learned a great deal from him about the vast and seemingly chaotic Medicaid program.

There are other books on Medicaid (e.g. Stevens and Stevens, 1974; and Holahan, 1975) written with different objectives. But this book delves as deeply as data and recorded experience permit into the mundane but extremely important matters of benefit levels, expenditure trends, utilization, payment methods, eligibility requirements, and legislative intent (or lack thereof). Davidson reveals how these bear heavily on beneficiaries and providers alike, and how they are related to the ambivalence of American society toward the poor, the apparent lack of faith in the integrity of the medical profession resulting in many rules governing all physicians in order to control a small minority, and equally onerous rules governing all beneficiaries, again to flush out a small minority. The book is as much an interpretation of American society and the politics of welfare as it is of the operation of Medicaid itself.

Odin W. Anderson, Ph.D.
University of Chicago
December 5, 1979

Preface

This is a book about Medicaid, the large federal-state program that pays for the medical care needed by certain categories of poor people. Several facts about Medicaid should be highlighted at the outset. For one thing, it is medicine *and* public welfare, and because it is affected by both systems the contribution of each needs to be understood. Second, like much activity in our complex contemporary society, it is an interorganizational program, not susceptible to the control of managers in any single bureaucratic hierarchy. It involves several components of the federal Department of Health and Human Services (formerly Health, Education and Welfare) which have not always worked closely together and it requires actions by governments at the federal, state, and sometimes the county levels. This last factor is related to a third characteristic of Medicaid, namely, that to a considerable extent it is not one program, but fifty, since the decisions that states make within the federally established framework of law and regulations determine the real character of the program.

The book is principally an analysis of the Medicaid expenditure problem which, simply put, is that dollar outlays have been growing at a substantial rate ever since the program was created in 1965 by the passage of Title XIX of the Social Security Act. State and federal governments have spent much of their effort in recent years trying to reduce these expenditures or at least to contain the rate of their increase. In that attempt the states have made decisions in several important areas, and it is a consideration of these decisions that forms the substance of the book.

In selecting the title *Medicaid Decisions,* I intended to call attention to actions taken by several important actors in the Medicaid drama. First among them are the states that determine the basic character of their programs by deciding who is to be covered, what services and how much of each they are to be covered for, how much providers of those services are to be paid and by what procedures, and how to monitor the program. Those decisions, in turn, affect decisions of the other two principal actors: the providers of services, most of whom can decide not only the extent of their participation but even whether they will participate at all, and the people who utilize services. The solution to the cost problem requires that the states make decisions that lead the providers and the users of services to act in ways that limit utilization and, thereby, expenditures without harming the health of the eligibles.

The analysis presented here is systematic in that it considers each decision area in detail and attempts to identify the contribution of each to solving the expenditure problem. This is done primarily by comparing the experience of the states according to the decisions they have made in each area. It is limited by the available data which, while they permit each topic to be discussed, do not allow either for considering the interaction of one with another or for controlling for the possible effects of other factors. Future studies may be able to correct this weakness as the data-generating capacities of state programs continue to improve.

It is hoped that this study represents a contribution to the field by virtue of three characteristics: first, it puts Medicaid into the context of state expenditures (Chapter 2); second, the conceptual approach that focuses on programmatic decisions at the state level, on the one hand, permits the effects of decisions in several important areas to be analyzed and, on the other, points the way to additional studies that can be planned to overcome the data limitations of the present work; and finally, the proposal presented in Chapter 8, while not new in all its particulars, is based firmly in the medical care literature and in the analysis presented in the previous chapters.

It is a pleasure for me to acknowledge with gratitude the help I have received during the several years that this project has been in progress. I am indebted to Deans Harold A. Richman and Margaret K. Rosenheim of the University of Chicago's School of Social Service Administration for the time I needed to carry out the study and for such a congenial working environment. The American Philosophical Society and the U. S. Administration on Aging provided generous financial suport.

In the collegial atmosphere of a great university it is not always possible to identify the many contributions of one's colleagues to a work of this type. I would be remiss, however, if I did not single out Elizabeth Kutza, Theodore Marmor, William Pollak, and John Schuerman not just for their assistance but equally for the graciousness with which they offered it. And I owe a particular debt to Odin W. Anderson, professor and director of the University's Center for Health Administration Studies, for many kindnesses over the years. It was Anderson, a distinguished medical care researcher, who first introduced me to the mysteries of Medicaid. He has continued to encourage and stimulate me, not the least by reading and commenting on the manuscript and by writing the Foreword to this volume.

I am also glad to have a chance to thank members and staff of the American Academy of Pediatrics who have given me the opportunity to test some of these ideas on them, thereby enriching my understanding of the reality in which public policies dependent on the private sector get implemented. I especially want to mention Doctors John P. Connelly, Donald W. Schiff, and George M. Wheatley, and Mr. Thomas P. Robb.

I have been fortunate to have had several research assistants at various stages of this project. They contributed not only their considerable energy, but also their ideas, a number of which can be found in the pages of the book. I am glad to be able to acknowledge in this small way my gratitude to Janet D. Perloff, Marsha S. Spear, David F. Gordon, and Michel Thibaut. In her careful editing, Susan Campbell helped me clarify a number of the points I was trying to make and increased the book's readability. Gwen Graham, Betty Bradley, and Danuta Sawicki helped by typing and preparing the manuscript for publication. None of these generous people is responsible for any errors that remain.

Finally, I want to thank my wife Harriet and our children Michael and Rachel for their continual support and encouragement throughout the length of this project, which finally has come to an end.

Stephen M. Davidson
Chicago, Illinois

Medicaid and Social Welfare

Medicaid is one of the several federal-state social welfare programs in which benefits are made available to eligible groups of citizens. In this case, the benefits are medical services, the eligibles are welfare recipients and the medically needy, and the mechanism is public payments to vendors of services. The first questions to ask are why should governments do this sort of thing—that is, why should they undertake social welfare programs? And, once having decided to have them, why do they employ the means chosen?

In this chapter I first discuss briefly the social welfare function in modern American society, both generally and in relation to medical care, and the choice between programs of universal entitlement and residual programs. Then I describe the Medicaid program which is the focus of this book.

THE SOCIAL WELFARE FUNCTION IN GOVERNMENT

Social welfare, according to Wolins, is "a device for maintaining or strengthening the existing social structure of an industrial society" (Wolins, 1967: 108). Why, we might ask, does the social structure need to be maintained or strengthened? Government intervenes to avert anticipated disruptions in the functioning of the society or to correct for them after they have occurred. But why is that necessary? Why does the society not perform these functions spontaneously?

In this country the answer lies in the fact that the United States is a political democracy with a capitalist economy. As a democracy, it rests on the principle that everyone is equal in the political process—

1

that everyone has one vote, a right to equal protection under the law, and the like. Yet the capitalist economy promotes inequality; in fact, it depends on it. Participants are guided by the understanding that a better idea and hard work will be rewarded with the money to purchase a better life: a more comfortable home, nicer clothes, more and better food, and leisure. And, since not everyone has equally valuable ideas or an equal capacity to work successfully at putting them into effect, those who do will acquire more than those who do not.

Okun calls this "the double standard of a capitalist democracy, professing and pursuing an egalitarian political and social system and simultaneously generating gaping disparities in economic well-being" (Okun, 1975: 1). This juxtaposition constitutes a problem in part because economic success may make one "more equal" in the political process. Economic winners are able to influence the outcomes of elections, for example, through their ability to contribute to a candidate's campaign for office. And, since most political leaders are lawyers and successful businessmen, well-to-do capitalists are likely to be part of the same social environment as political officials and, therefore, to have easier access to them than working people. Thus economic inequality leads to political inequality, and, if it is played out to its logical conclusion, it could lead to the erosion of the political rights on which the society rests. The results might be that the government created to preserve and protect the society might end up preserving and protecting the economic elite at the expense of the economically least successful.

Some theorists believe that this is as it should be. They believe that potential economic reward drives citizens to ever greater effort in the hopes of achieving higher incomes and the comforts they can buy. Taking that potential away, they argue, would result in the erosion of ambition and aspiration and the initiative they foster; giving the losers that which they have not won would undermine the very principles of the progress on which the economy depends. Yet, others contend, letting the forces that produce inequality proceed unchecked to their ultimate conclusions would undermine the political foundation on which the economic structure is built.

Of course, even a substantial amount of economic inequality might be tolerable as long as a society remained mobile and people in lower economic strata could realistically aspire to advance. Evidence is plentiful, however, to demonstrate that the share of wealth owned by the lowest fifth of the population that has in fact declined over the past seventy-five years. So, even though the middle class may be becoming more secure economically, the lower economic groups are becoming more firmly entrenched in the depths. The poorest among us apparently are systematically denied the opportunity to move up the ladder of economic success—access to education, for example, a critical ticket to advancement, is blocked. While the outward measures of success are present—high-school graduates are increasing—the value of those statistics is diminished by the growing numbers of high-school graduates who read and write so poorly as to be virtually illiterate.

In the past forty years the interventionists have won many battles, and the result is a growing number of social welfare programs aimed at reducing the inequalities produced by the rampant opportunism inherent in unchecked capitalism. But the decisions leading to these programs were not the result solely of the altruism borne of compassion for human suffering. As Wolins says, "while love of one's fellow man may have been a motive for some individual reformers and welfare leaders . . . it has not been the force that has moved men in power" (Wolins, 1967; 108). They have acted, instead, largely out of self-interest. They perceive that when inequality is too great, poverty too common, and the capitalist's dream too far out of reach to offer the poor anything but despair, the economic and social order that is of such benefit to the successful in business and the professions is threatened. If those on the bottom rungs of the economic ladder become desperate to survive, they may lash out, even violently, at the order that they blame for their plight. Thus, the winners have some stake in cutting the losses of the losers. The result is social welfare policy—public policy that gives medical care, social services, housing, education, and even cash to people unable to obtain them for themselves.

Okun describes the problem as a tradeoff between the efficiency promoted by the free market system and the equality necessary for the functioning of democracy. One of "the ways in which American society promotes equality (and pays some costs in terms of efficiency) is by establishing social and political rights that are distributed equally and universally and . . . are intended to be kept out of the market place" (Okun, 1975: 4). A large and growing number of "entitlements and privileges are distributed universally and equally and free of charge to all adult citizens of the United States" (1975: 6). Among the principal attributes of rights are that they "are acquired and exercised without any monetary charge"; do not encourage people to specialize in things they do well in order to obtain an advantage; are distributed not "as incentives, or as rewards and penalties," but rather equally, "even at the expense of equity and freedom," and cannot be bought or sold (1975: 6–10).

The list of rights, which has been expanding in the United States in this century, includes items that seriously affect the ability of citizens to participate in the life of the society, and the absence of which might undermine the viability of the society. Thus, minimal Social Security benefits in one's retirement have become a right (since 1966 people have been entitled to benefits at age seventy-two even if they have not contributed to the system). This development resulted in part from humanitarian recognition of the need for income in one's old age and in part from a desire to protect the society as growing numbers survive beyond the age at which they can contribute productively to the economy (though obviously some are able to work longer than others) and as families are unavailable or unable to support such persons. Their purchasing power (and, thus, a part of their ability to contribute to the economy) is preserved, and they are not penalized for being without a family that can reabsorb them. Indeed, Okun even argues that "the principle of contribution serves mainly to preserve pride," not to finance the program (1975: 19).

Other services recognized as important are distributed to some citizens through government intervention even though they have not yet been accorded the status of rights. Medical care is such a service, and, if a national health insurance program becomes law, it may one day become a right. Indeed, in the early 1970s the argument was often heard that citizens had a right to medical care (if not to health). The importance of public intervention to insure access to medical care—as well as the case for adding this area to the expanding list of rights—rests on the necessity of good health for survival and for productivity, the assumed connection (more and more frequently challenged of late) between medical care and health, and observed deficits in the utilization of services on the part of the poor and the elderly in particular.

Students cannot learn if they are absent from school because of ill health; workers cannot support their families if they are unable to keep their jobs because of ill health. And good health is not distributed randomly throughout the population.

Data from the Health Interview Survey of the National Center for Health Statistics before the passage of Medicare and Medicaid confirmed this truth. In Table 1-1 it can be seen that more often than not the poor had higher rates of chronic conditions, acute conditions, and disability days than other income groups. Further, the extent of the problem tended to increase with age. Thus, the lowest income groups were 15.7 percent and 10.2 percent more likely to have chronic conditions than the highest groups of adults forty-five through sixty-four and sixty-five or older, respectively, in 1962 and 1963. The figures showing the incidence of acute conditions per one hundred persons for those two age groups were even more dramatic. These figures, moreover, probably understated the true extent of acute illness since they excluded conditions for which no medical attention was sought or which did not result in restricted activity. Data on disability days per person per year reveal a still clearer pattern, although age was not considered there. In every type of disability reported, the lowest income groups experienced considerably more disability than the highest income groups.

Table 1-1.   Health and Income, 1962-1963

	Income			
	Under $2,000	$2,000— 3,999	$4,000— 6,999	$7,000 or More
A. Percent of Population with One or More Chronic Conditions, by Family Income and Age				
Age				
Under 15 years	19.2	19.4	18.8	20.8
15–44 years	48.3	45.3	46.2	46.6
45–64 years	76.8	68.3	62.3	61.1
65 or more years	86.4	81.4	77.2	76.2
B. Incidence of Acute Conditions per 100 Persons per Year, by Family Income and Age[a]				
Age				
Under 15 years	259.0	264.8	302.4	349.8
15–44 years	208.1	200.0	199.4	203.8
45–64 years	187.3	153.9	149.4	162.6
65 or more years	162.8	125.8	136.1	101.5
C. Disability Days per Person per Year, by Family Income				
Restricted activity days	29.1	17.7	13.7	13.1
Bed disability days	12.0	7.4	5.6	5.2
School-loss days	6.5	5.1	5.3	5.8
Work-loss days	8.9	7.3	5.8	5.4

Source: U.S. National Center for Health Statistics, *Medical Care, Health Status, and Family Income,* Vital and Health Statistics, Series 10, Number 9, Washington, D.C.: USDHEW, 1964, pp. 53, 67, 70.

[a]Excludes conditions involving neither restricted activity nor medical attention.

Not only was good health not equally distributed in the society, but also the groups with the greatest need were among the least able to pay for the medical care that can correct for illness. These facts are reflected in figures for the period which show that utilization increased with income (see Table 1-2).

Table 1–2. Utilization of Physician and Hospital Services, by Income, 1963–1964

Family Income	Number Physician Visits per Person per Year[a]	Percent of People with One or More Physician Visits in Past Year[b]	Hospital Discharges per 1,000 People per Year[c]	Average Length of Stay[d]
Under $2,000	4.3	59.2	136.4	10.2
$2,000–3,999	4.3	61.9	145.6	9.4
$4,000–6,999	4.5	66.3	128.0	7.2
$7,000–9,999	4.7	69.8	121.7	7.2
$10,000 or more	5.1	72.8	116.5	7.4

Percent of People with Selected Symptoms Seeing a Physician within a Year by Income, 1963[e]

Family Income	Percent Getting Up Tired	Percent Sore Throat, Fever	Percent Waking Up with Stiff Joints	Percent with Frequent Headaches	Percent with Sudden Weakness or Faintness	Percent with Frequent Backaches
Low	31	46	30	33	50	42
Middle	32	61	30	42	54	45
High	31	67	34	43	57	45

[a] National Center for Health Statistics, Volume of Physician Visits by Place of Visit and Type of Service, Vital and Health Statistics, Series 10, Number 18, Washington, D.C.: USDHEW, 1965, p. 19.
[b] National Center for Health Statistics, Physician Visits, Interval of Visits and Children's Routine Checkup, Vital and Health Statistics, Series 10, Number 19, Washington, D.C.: USDHEW, 1965, p. 24.
[c] National Center for Health Statistics, Hospital Discharges and Length of Stay: Short-Stay Hospitals, Vital and Health Statistics, Series 10, Number 30, Washington, D.C.: USDHEW, 1966, p. 36.
[d] Ibid., p. 37.
[e] Andersen, Lion, Anderson, 1976:24.

The lowest income were least likely to have seen a physician in the previous year and, among those who did see physicians, they were likely to have had the fewest visits (see Table 1–2). Moreover, Andersen, Lion, and Anderson (1976: 24) showed that for each of several symptoms considered, the lowest income groups were generally least likely to have sought the services of physicians. That is, they put off seeking medical attention which people with higher incomes received. The poor were more likely to have been hospitalized than other income groups, but their longer average length of stay indicated that the conditions for which they were admitted to hospitals were more serious.

So, in 1965, when Medicare and Medicaid became law as Titles XVIII and XIX of the Social Security Act, there was much evidence to demonstrate that the poor and elderly were more likely to need medical services than others and less likely to be able to pay for them. Having decided at that time that a public benefit existed in making medical care easier to obtain for people who had systematically had difficulty in getting it,[a] the public officials who created the programs had several questions to consider in designing them:

1. Who should be covered? All or only those in need?
2. How should they be covered? Through universal or means-tested criteria?
3. What services and how much of each should be covered?
4. Where should they get the services? In special centers or in the mainstream?

The developers of many social welfare programs have faced these questions, and their resolution not only reveals deep-seated attitudes about government and about the needy but also determines to a considerable degree the operation of the programs following passage.

In the United States the role of government in medical care has historically been limited to providing assistance to special groups. This tendency began with the creation of the Public Health Service for the benefit of merchant seamen in the eighteenth century and continued through the mid-1960s programs for the poor and elderly (e.g., Medicare, Medicaid, Neighborhood Health Centers; see Anderson, 1968). It has been assumed that medical care is a commodity that can be purchased by most people in need of it and that there are benefits to be gained from letting the medical care market respond to that private demand for services. Indeed, much of that attitude remains today and serves as a major obstacle to the enactment of national health insurance for all Americans. The only exception to date has been some of the efforts at containing medical care expenditures. Certificate-of-need laws enacted in many states, for example, apply to all hospitals contemplating capital expenditures of a designated amount, often $100,000. Professional Standards Review Organiza-

[a] In addition to the public benefit, elected public officials perceived political benefits in the passage of Medicare and Medicaid. For a good discussion of the events leading to the passage of this legislation, see Marmor (1973).

tions (PSROs), on the other hand, are more in keeping with that tradition. They are designed to monitor utilization only by beneficiaries of the programs in the Social Security Act (Medicare, Medicaid, or the children's programs under Title V).

While these policies are defensible in historical and political terms and on the basis of certain economic theories, "universalism in social welfare . . . [is] a needed prerequisite towards reducing and removing formal barriers of social and economic discrimination" (Titmuss, 1967: 196—97). Universalism, in this sense, is the provision of social welfare services, including medical care, to all in the society without discrimination against any. A national health insurance plan under which all citizens were eligible would be a universal program; a program that applies only to some of the poor is not. To the extent that a program serves only some groups—even if the intent is compensatory—it sanctions discrimination between the eligibles and others.[b]

However, the principle of universalism can be applied even when the goal is to compensate for poverty. Social Security and Medicare in the United States are examples. These institutional programs rest on the assumption that old age is a period of limited income, and they further assume that these incomes need to be raised and that old people must be able to purchase needed medical services. Instead of testing the income of individual elderly persons, however, these programs assume that all of the elderly have need to some extent. Therefore, to establish eligibility for benefits all one need do is demonstrate that one has reached the required age (and, in some cases for Social Security, contributed to the trust funds in earlier years). Eligibility is automatic for such people; they do not have to demonstrate that they in fact are poor. Welfare and Medicaid, its medical care component, are, in contrast, residual programs. They require that individual applicants for benefits demonstrate not only that they are poor but also that they meet certain other requirements (which vary with the state). Clearly, it is more of a burden to establish eligibility under residual programs than under institutional ones. I return to this issue in Chapter 4.

Some American medical care programs provide funds for the purchase of services in the private sector (Medicare and Medicaid), and others establish special services to meet the needs of groups for whom financial capacity is not the only barrier to the utilization of needed services (e.g., the National Health Service Corps places physi-

---

[b] Theoretically, it may be possible for such a program to make conditions for the poor even better than those existing in the market-place for the rest of society, but that has never been the case in our history. Separate programs usually are inferior ones.

cians and other personnel in remote sites deficient in medical care resources; the Rural Health Clinics Act permits nurse practitioners to provide services under certain conditions in areas without physicians; and Neighborhood Health Centers and Children and Youth Programs have been established in other areas lacking in services, notably inner cities). On the one hand, programs providing for the purchase of medical services in the private sector have the potential of integrating poor people and others in need into the mainstream of American medicine and avoid the expense of creating complex new organizations to provide services. Special programs, on the other hand, are useful when there are innovations to be tested. Also, private sector programs are generally able to reach more people because their impact is not limited to the locations in which the special programs are established to provide services.

Medicaid, the subject of the analysis presented in the following chapters, is an example of a means-tested, residual welfare program. Because it makes use of the private sector, it has the potential of reaching more people than the special programs. But, because it is a residual program, one intended to pick up the slack when the market and the family do not meet the need, it has restricted eligibility (see Wilensky and Lebeaux, 1958). As such, it has some of the characteristics of the welfare system and some of the medical care system, and it is important to understand something of both in order to do a thorough analysis.[c]

THE MEDICAID PROGRAM

Medicaid was created by Title XIX of the Social Security Act, passed in 1965 along with Title XVIII, Medicare, the national health insurance program for the elderly (see Marmor, 1973; Somers and Somers, 1967; and Stevens and Stevens, 1974, for discussions of the passage of these two laws). Under its terms, federal funds were made available to the states to help pay the cost of medical care purchased on behalf of eligible poor people. One goal was to make medical care accessible in the mainstream of American medicine to eligible poor people to an extent never before achieved. It was to be the means of integrating them fully into the private medical care system in the United States. Several points which will be referred to throughout the analysis should be highlighted in this introduction to the Medicaid program: the range of services covered; the program's relation to the welfare system; federal and state roles in the program; variations

[c] A brief discussion of the medical care system is found in Chapter 3.

among state programs; and Medicaid's record of genuine accomplishment.

Covered Services

To participate in Medicaid, states were required to develop a state plan with certain characteristics, one of which was the coverage of at least five basic services: inpatient hospital services, outpatient hospital services, physicians' services, laboratory and X-ray services, and nursing home services. Subsequent amendments required early and periodic screening, diagnosis, and treatment services for eligible children (EPSDT) and family planning services, and permitted payments for services in intermediate care facilities (in addition to the skilled nursing facilities required by the original law). If the state program provided for the medically indigent (see the next section), any seven of fifteen enumerated services were to be included for them. These were minimum standards; virtually any additional health care service recognized by a state could also be included.

Since each state developed its own plan, it is not surprising to find that, within these limits, the states vary considerably in the services they make available to cligible residents. (These differences and their implications are discussed in more detail in Chapters 5 and 8.) States may differ from one another both in the range of services included and in the amount of each for which payment will be made. For example, some states limit their programs to the services mandated by federal law, while other states include virtually all health care services available in their states. Thus, dental services may be covered in some states and not in others; similarly, physical therapy, optometric, and podiatric services are available to eligibles in only some states. Moreover, some states make available to categorically eligible clients (that is, welfare recipients) a different list of services than they make available to the medically needy (people who share the characteristics of welfare recipients except that they have incomes of up to 133.3 percent of the maximum amount paid to recipients of Aid to Families with Dependent Children).

Furthermore, variation occurs even within the range of mandated services. In some states, clients are eligible for an unlimited number of physician visits in a year; in others, they are restricted to one visit a month. Some states pay for necessary hospitalizations without any limit in length; others pay for a maximum of, for example, twenty days in a year. One implication of these variations is inequity among welfare recipients from state to state. A Medicaid eligible in St. Louis, Missouri, for example, is entitled to many fewer services than a resident of East St. Louis, across the Mississippi River in Illinois.

Another is that it makes assessments of Medicaid as a national program quite difficult.

Relation to Welfare

The public welfare system in the United States is, like Medicaid, a federal/state program. The federal government establishes certain minimal criteria and pays part of the bill, but the states develop their own plans within those guidelines and administer the program (i.e., determine client eligibility, issue cash grants, and provide services). Public welfare is a means-tested cash assistance program that provides cash grants to eligible poor people in four categories: aged, blind, disabled, and families with dependent children (AFDC). In 1974, the first three categories (the adult categories) were federalized under the Supplemental Security Income (SSI) program.[d] AFDC remains a federal/state program. This discussion is relevant because all AFDC recipients and most SSI recipients are eligible for Medicaid benefits by virtue of their welfare status.

Eligibility, which again is primarily a state function (there is variation even in the federal SSI categories), depends on applicant income and resources and family characteristics. Thus, the income level for eligibility varies from state to state, and so do the rules about other assets (e.g., homes, cars, other personal property), including, in some cases, rules for disposing of property. Also, the program tends to penalize families for their completeness. In many states, a family with a father is ineligible for benefits until the father leaves, even if the father is unemployed or employed at a job in which he earns less than the eligibility level of income. In other states, however, families with fathers are eligible for benefits.

Moreover, since welfare eligibility depends on family income, there must be periodic redeterminations of eligibility (as often as monthly), and a welfare family whose head is able to secure a job is penalized by the loss of the cash grant and Medicaid benefits as soon as the employment becomes known to the state welfare department. To a considerable extent, therefore, the welfare program contains disincentives for families trying to become economically self-sufficient because it fails to recognize that the jobs available to poorly educated recipients are generally low paying and unstable. These issues are beyond the scope of the present analysis, but they are relevant to Medicaid because they mean that many welfare families are headed by women (which has implications for the utilization of medical services); because they may cause eligibility for medical benefits to change from month to month, thus interfering, potentially at least,

---

[d]The states retain a role in SSI, particularly regarding eligibility for Medicaid. See Chapter 5.

with the recipients' ability to receive continuing medical care; and because they raise issues of equity.

Federal and State Roles

As noted above, the federal government establishes the ground rules for Medicaid and pays part of the bill; the states define the program within the limits of those regulations, pay the rest of the bill, and administer the program. Because federal officials are concerned primarily with the extent to which the states follow the federal rules and with the level of programmatic expenditures, they monitor the state programs by requiring periodic reports of activities, and they institute policies and programs designed to contain Medicaid expenditures.

Thus, the federal government has required that each state establish a Medicaid Management Information System (MMIS), a claims-based computerized data collection and analysis capability. Some states have been slow to adopt this system, but in recent years the numbers with approved MMISs have increased to the point that more than half the states now have them in place. It is not clear, however, to what extent they are actually used to monitor the programs, identify problem areas and trends, and inform the states' policymaking processes.

Federal law now also requires Professional Standards Review Organizations (PSROs), associations of physicians at the state level (or, in some large states, at the level of subareas within states) that monitor and control the utilization of Medicaid services. These organizations (described in more detail in Chapter 7) have concentrated their activities on hospital services, but their mandate extends to all services and the expectation is that they will expand their operations to nursing homes, physicians and other providers of care.

The states are charged with administering Medicaid. They establish eligibility criteria and procedures, enroll clients and participating providers, pay claims for services rendered, monitor the operation of the program, and are responsible for its integrity. Some of the decisions taken to perform these functions are discussed in subsequent chapters, particularly in the context of their implications for program expenditures.

Variations among the States

I have already indicated some of the ways in which Medicaid varies from state to state: number of services covered, amount of each service covered, and eligibility. Other areas in which variations can be observed are the adoption, implementation, and use of MMISs, and the rules and rates for paying bills.

States are required to pay hospitals and nursing homes on the ba-sis of their costs, using complex rules described in considerable detail in the Code of Federal Regulations (see Chapter 5). They are re-quired to pay other providers on the basis of their charges. In neither case is it true, however, that the program pays the providers all that the providers believe they are entitled to receive. Thus, while institu-tional services are pegged to costs, the definition of legitimate costs varies with the state and so does the proportion of costs (however they are defined) actually paid. Hospitals may receive 70 percent of their costs for example. Physicians or other professionals may be paid, not the full amount charged to the program or to non-Medicaid patients, but the least of their billed charges, their profile of charges for a particular service, and the prevailing charges in the area. More-over, payment may be pegged at the seventieth percentile of the pre-vailing charge. Finally, for both institutional and professional providers, the rates may be revised infrequently and, thus, not keep up with the increasing cost of doing business. (The New York State fee schedule for physicians, for example, has not been revised since 1968.) These state policies are governed primarily by state preoccu-pation with increasing Medicaid expenditures (see Chapter 2), for it is true that, even though providers complain bitterly about low rates of pay and inefficient, unpredictable payment methods, the amounts of services provided have generally been increasing and so have state outlays for those services.

The extent to which Medicaid programs vary from state to state has been captured dramatically by a measure called the Medicaid Program Index (MPI; see Davidson, 1978). The MPI is a summary measure calculated from data on four important aspects of variability in state Medicaid programs: eligibility of the medically indigent for benefits, the number of optional services covered, limitations placed on the provision of the basic services, and reimbursement procedures. It is computed according to the procedures summarized in Table 1–3.

That the state Medicaid programs do indeed vary can be seen from the scores on the MPI components for 1975 displayed in Table 1–4. The totals range from 8 to 13, as summarized in Table 1–5. Since, as indicated by the MPI, the states vary in important program charac-teristics it is possible to analyze the cost problem by comparing states that have adopted one policy with states that have adopted another. (This is the basis of the analysis presented in Chapters 2 through 7.) The MPI also reveals a weakness of this method, howev-er; there are changes over time that it cannot take into account (see Davidson, 1978). Between 1970 and 1975, for example, there were substantial changes, reflected in the MPI scores, that generally had the effect of liberalizing the state programs (Davidson, 1978). There is some evidence, as yet unpublished, to suggest that, since then, there have been changes in the opposite direction. Moreover, while the MPI is undoubtedly useful for describing interstate variations at a single point and in comparing them at several points, its utility as an analytic tool has yet to be demonstrated.[c]

Table 1-3.   Calculation of the Program Index

Dimension	Conditions		Coded Score
(1) Medically indigent	Not included in program		1
	Included in program		2
(2) Optional services	Number provided:	0	0
		1–4	1
		5–9	2
		10–14	3
		15–	4
(3) Limitations on provision of services	For each basic service if there are:		
	Limits and prior authorization required	=0	
	Limits but no prior authorization required or		
	No limits but prior authorization is required	=1	
	No limits and no prior authorization	=2	
	If the total score for all five basic services combined is:	0 Then	0
		1–2	1
		3–5	2
		6–8	3
		9–10	4
(4) Reimbursement procedures	For each basic service, if reimbursement is based on:		
	Fee schedule	=0	
	Reasonable cost ⎫ Maximum cost/unit time ⎬	=1	
	Percentage of charges ⎫ Negotiated charge ⎪ Reasonable charge ⎬ Usual and customary charge ⎪ with a maximum ⎭	=2	
	Usual and customary charge	=3	
	If the total score for all five basic services combined is:	0 Then	0
		1–3	1
		4–7	2
		8–11	3
		12–	4
Medicaid Program Index	A final score for the Medicaid Program Index was obtained by adding the coded scores for each of the four dimensions.		

Source: Davidson (1978b).

[c] A test of it is now under way as part of a study by the American Academy of Pediatrics on "Variations by State in Physician Participation in the Medicaid Programs." The research is being supported by the Health Care Financing Administration (Grant No. 18-P-97159/5).

Table 1-4.   Components of the Medicaid Program Index, 1975

	Inclusion of Medically Needy	Optional Services	Limitations	Reimbursement Procedures	Total MPI
	1975	1975	1975	1975	1975
Alabama		2	3	3	9
Alaska		2	4	3	10
Arizona		1	4		6
Arkansas	x	3	3	2	10
California	x	4	3	3	12
Colorado		2	4	3	10
Connecticut	x	4	3	2	11
Delaware		2	4	2	9
D.C.	x	3	4	2	11
Florida		2	3	2	8
Georgia		3	4	2	10
Hawaii	x	3	2	3	10
Idaho		2	4	3	10
Illinois	x	4	4	3	13
Indiana		3	4	3	11
Iowa	x	4	4	3	13
Kansas	x	4	4	2	12
Kentucky	x	3	2	2	9
Louisiana		3	3	3	10
Maine	x	4	4	2	12
Maryland	x	3	3	1	9
Massachusetts	x	4	4	2	12
Michigan	x	4	4	2	12
Minnesota	x	4	4	3	13
Mississippi		2	3	2	8
Missouri		2	3	3	9
Montana	x	4	3	3	12
Nebraska	x	4	4	2	12
Nevada		4	3	2	10
New Hampshire	x	3	3	2	10
New Jersey		4	3	3	11
New Mexico		3	4	3	11
New York	x	4	4	2	12
North Carolina	x	3	4	2	11
North Dakota	x	4	4	3	13
Ohio		4	4	3	12
Oklahoma	x	2	3	3	10
Oregon		4	4	1	10
Pennsylvania	x	3	3	1	9
Rhode Island	x	2	3	1	9
South Carolina		4	4	2	11
South Dakota		3	4	4	10
Tennessee	x	2	3	2	9
Texas		3	4	3	11
Utah	x	4	4	3	13
Vermont	x	3	3	2	10
Virginia	x	3	4	2	11
Washington	x	4	3	1	10
West Virginia	x	4	4	1	11
Wisconsin	x	4	4	3	13
Wyoming		1	4	3	9

Source: Davidson (1978b)

Table 1–5. Summary Results of Medicaid Program Index, 1975

Score	Number of States
8	2
9	9
10	13
11	10
12	9
13	6

Source: Table 1–4.

Accomplishments of Medicaid

While any program as complex as Medicaid can be expected to generate problems, and though much of the analysis of Medicaid by students of public policy focuses on those problems, it should be made clear that Medicaid has had the effect of increasing the utilization of health care services by the poor, just as it was intended to do (see, for example, Davis and Schoen, 1978; and Andersen, Lion, and Anderson, 1976). Table 1–6 when compared with Table 1–2, shows the gains made by poor people in utilization of services. The almost linear relationship between income and utilization observed in the early 1960s prior to the program has been reversed, so that now, in many instances, the poor use more services than wealthier Americans. Since the poor have greater need for services because of their greater incidence of illness and the tendency for their illnesses to be more severe than those of others, the reversal is cause for pride that a public program has had the desired effect.

Nonetheless, there is evidence to suggest that deficits remain (see Davis and Schoen, 1978, for example), especially for some groups of poor people. Moreover, some of the monitoring programs indicate that there is unnecessary utilization by poor and nonpoor alike. That the program has achieved some measure of success is indicated by the fact that much effort now is being directed to reducing its costs (the result of increased utilization) and that attention to redressing the remaining deficiencies in utilization has diminished.

It is the problem of costs that is the principal focus of this volume. Medicaid costs have indeed increased substantially over the years since the program's enactment in the mid-1960s, to the point that many consider it to be the principal public policy problem in the area of health care. A number of measures to reduce expenditures have been taken in the past several years. In this book I examine and assess these Medicaid decisions. After describing the cost problem and placing it in context in Chapter 2, I discuss some of the sources of the increased expenditures and some of the attemps to reduce them in Chapters 3 through 7. The particular topics chosen (eligibility, benefits, provider compensation, and monitoring) were selected because of their presumed role in the cost problem and because they are in large part decisions taken at the state level. Further, since state programs vary because of decisions on those issues, it is possible to compare expenditure levels and rates among the states according to their positions on each of those questions. Finally, in Chapter 8, I offer a proposal designed to moderate the level of Medicaid expenditures while continuing to improve the program's record of accomplishments.

Table 1–6. Utilization of Physician and Hospital Services, by Income, 1972 and 1973

Family Income		Number Physician Visits per Person per Year, 1973	Percent of People with One or More Physician Visits in Past Year, 1973	Hospital Discharges per 1,000 People per Year, 1972	Average Length of Stay, 1972
Lowest	1	6.0	74.7	185.4	10.5
	2	5.5	73.1	149.1	9.7
	3	4.9	71.4	130.6	8.3
	4	4.8	73.9	116.6	7.3
	5	4.9	75.3	103.3	6.8
Highest	6	—	77.4	—	—

Sources: U.S. National Center for Health Statistics, Vital and Health Statistics, Series 10, Number 97, p. 5 (physicians) and unpublished data (hospital).

The Cost of Medicaid

2

The cost of Medicaid has attracted more public attention than any other aspect of the program. Medicaid expenditures have been growing at a substantial rate annually since the program's inception. Initially, at least, the rate of growth was unexpected, and that highlighted a central problem of planning: how to anticipate expenditures more accurately. On another level, the sheer amount of the expenditures, particularly at the state level, has strained public budgets. It is this problem that is the principal focus of this chapter.

The problem can be seen in the following simple equation:

$$\text{Medicaid expenditures} = \text{volume of services used by eligibles} \times \text{price of services}$$

A public policy question has arisen because the left side of the equation has grown at a considerable rate, thereby forcing states to raise additional revenues for the program. As expenditures have increased to the point at which they exert pressure on other decision-making centers (e.g., tax policy and competing programs), attempts have been made to reduce the numbers on the right side of the equation in order to reduce the total expenditures.

To maintain the equation in balance, any of its members can be altered. For example, the amount of money to spend can be increased by raising taxes, by diverting funds from other public uses, or both. Alternatively, the volume of services can be reduced by limiting one or more of the following: the numbers of people who are eligible to receive services, the numbers of people or institutions authorized to provide services, the types of services that are covered, and the amounts of services that will be paid for (either by limiting the amounts of services covered or by attempting to control the utilization of covered services through devices like Professional Standards Review Organizations). Finally, the state can limit the price it is willing to pay for services.

Since the volume of services used is determined by multiplying the number of users by the rate of use, the equation can be elaborated as follows:

$$\text{Medicaid expenditures} = \text{number of users} \times \text{rate of use} \times \text{price}$$

Moreover, the right side of the equation must be calculated for each type of covered service. The full equation can thus be written as follows:

$$\text{Medicaid expenditures} = (\text{number of users of physician services} \times \text{rate of use of physician services} \times \text{price of physician services}) + (\text{number of users of hospital services} \times \text{rate of use of hospital services} \times \text{price of hospital services}) + (\text{number of users of service C} \times \text{rate of use of service C} \times \text{price of service C}) + \ldots + (\text{number of users of service N} \times \text{rate of use of service N} \times \text{Price of service N})$$

Thus, in order to understand fully the growth in Medicaid expenditures, it is necessary to examine (1) the users of each service, (2) the rates of use of each service, and (3) the price of each service. Furthermore, since the number of users of each service is, to a considerable extent a reflection of the numbers of people eligible for Medicaid benefits, (Holahan, 1975), the analysis must include a consideration of trends in Medicaid eligibility as well. In this chapter the several parts of the equation will be examined, first to define the extent of the problem and then to explain the growth in expenditures. (A similar treatment of the utilization of services is presented in the next chapter.)

Table 2-1. Expenditures For Medical Vendor Payments, 1965–1977[a]

In Millions of Dollars

	1965	1966	1967	1968	1969	1970	1971	1972	1973	1974	1975	1976	1977[b]
Total	1,479	2,040	2,944	4,254	4,871	5,745	7,015	8,480	10,214	10,372	13,915	15,437	17,620
Federal share	632	961	1,587	2,114	2,436	2,990	3,770	4,582	5,411	5,833	7,428	8,597	9,713
State and local share	847	1,079	1,357	2,140	2,435	2,755	3,245	3,898	4,803	4,539	6,487	6,841	7,906

In Percent

	1965	1966	1967	1968	1969	1970	1971	1972	1973	1974	1975	1976	1977[b]
Total	100.0	100.0	100.0	100.0	100.0	100.0	100.0	100.0	100.0	100.0	100.0	100.0	100.0
Federal share	42.7	47.1	53.9	49.7	50.0	52.0	53.7	54.0	53.0	56.2	53.4	55.7	55.1
State and local share	57.3	52.9	46.1	50.3	50.0	48.0	46.3	46.0	47.0	43.8	46.6	44.3	44.9

Percent Change

	1965–66	1966–67	1967–68	1968–69	1969–70	1970–71	1971–72	1972–73	1973–74	1974–75	1975–76	1976–77
Total	37.9	44.3	44.5	14.5	17.9	22.1	20.9	20.4	1.5	34.2	10.9	14.1
Federal share	52.1	65.1	33.2	15.2	22.7	26.1	21.5	18.1	7.8	27.3	15.7	13.0
State and local share	27.4	25.8	57.7	13.8	13.1	17.8	20.1	23.2	-5.5	42.9	5.3	15.6

Sources: B.S. Cooper et al., *Compendium of National Health Expenditures Data*, ORS/SSA/DHEW, Pub. No. (SSA) 76–11927, January 1976, table 9.

R.M. Gibson and M.S. Mueller, National Health Expenditures, Fiscal Year 1976, *Social Security Bulletin*, April 1977, pp. 3—22.

R.M. Gibson and C.R. Fisher, National Health Expenditures, Fiscal Year 1977, *Social Security Bulletin*, July 1978, pp. 3—20.

[a]Totals include Guam, Puerto Rico, and the Virgin Islands.
[b]Preliminary estimates.

MEDICAID EXPENDITURES

Total expenditures on Medical Vendor Payments increased from $1,479,000,000 in 1965, before Medicaid became effective, to $15,437,000,000 in 1976 (see Table 2–1). The intervening eleven years saw expenditures grow by almost $14 billion, or almost 1,000 percent. While the program caused public expenditures to mushroom, it also distributed that large new burden differently between federal and nonfederal public sources. The state and local share of medical vendor payments amounted to 57 percent of the total in 1965 and to only 44 percent by 1976. Yet, while the state and local proportional share was falling, their share in actual dollars rose by almost $6 billion during that period, a 708 percent increase. During the same period, the federal share increased by 1,260 percent, or almost $8 billion.

At the same time that public expenditures for medical vendor payments were increasing by almost 1,000 percent, the states were increasing their expenditures in other areas as well (see Table A–1). Several points are worth noting.

1. Public welfare expenditures increased by more than $24 billion, amounting to a gain of almost 450 percent. Medical vendor payments grew from 27 percent of welfare expenditures to 52 percent. Thus, while the medical portion of welfare costs was growing by almost 950 percent, the nonmedical portion was increasing by only 260 percent, more than a threefold difference.
2. Public welfare's share of total state expenditures grew by 4.4 percent. Education, after a larger increase, began to decline, so that its share was only 0.9 percent higher in 1976 than it had been in 1965.
3. The proportion of state expenditures for highways dropped by 11.7 percent. The amount spent for welfare, which began the period as 55 percent of highway expenditures, actually surpassed highway costs, so that by 1976, it was 164 percent of highway money.

Thus, of the three items examined, public welfare's rate of growth, including Medicaid, was higher than any of the others. It grew by almost 450 percent, while education expenditures increased by 310 percent and those for highways by only 84 percent. Total state expenditures grew by 300 percent.

Even though medical vendor payments increased nine and one-half times and all welfare expenditures, four and one-half times, total state costs increased by only three times. By 1976 welfare still accounted for less than one-fifth of state expenditures, while education represented more than one-third of state outlays. State government in general was expanding, and although the welfare component was growing faster than others, its relative magnitude was still such that other sectors of state government accounted for 82 percent of the total growth.

Another aspect of the financial burden of Medicaid is the distribution of program costs among federal, state, and local sources. While it is not possible, given present data sources, to apportion nonfederal Medicaid costs among local and state governments, it is possible to do it with other services and to make some inferences about Medicaid.

Table A–2 presents the distribution of state revenues from federal and local governments for several purposes. From those data we can see that the local share of public welfare expenditures rose astronomically during the period from 1965 through 1976. Overall, state revenues from other governments increased by more than 333 percent and those for education and public welfare grew by 515 percent and 452 percent, respectively.

Referring to Table A–1, we can see that the only category for which nonstate revenues did not increase substantially faster than state revenues was highways. In other words, even though state expenditures overall and for education and welfare in particular increased at a substantial rate during the period, the burden of those increases fell on other levels of government more heavily than on the states themselves.

This point is made explicit in Table A–3 which presents state revenues used for the three purposes we have been considering and for total state expenditures. It shows that the states themselves had to raise 290 percent more money in 1976 than they raised in 1965. Public welfare required more than the general increase, education about the same, and highways less.

Looking at the actual dollars raised completes the context (see Tables A–3 and A–4). Of the $102 billion that states needed in 1976 over their requirements in 1965, 37 percent of the increase went for education, while only 9.7 percent was needed for public welfare. Moreover, in actual dollars, the highway requirement was only 4 percent less than that for welfare.

Table 2–1 showed that the combined state and local share for medical vendor payments grew by only $5,994 million. Thus, comparing data in Tables 2–1 and A–3, we can infer—without, however, being able to identify the amounts precisely—that the state share of medical vendor payments increased by about the same amount as the state share of highway expenditures (i.e., $5,994 million versus $5,878 million).

None of this is meant to deny the large proportional increases in medical vendor payments during this period nor to imply that they have not had an important effect on state budgets and on medical expenditures and even on the medical care system generally. It might also be argued that an investment in highways contributes more to the economy of a state than equivalent outlays for welfare or welfare-connected medical services. It is worth pointing out, however, that in real terms, highways have increased the states' financial burden as much as medical vendor payments, notwithstanding the fact that this point is obscured by accounts in the public press that have focused primarily on Medicaid increases.[a]

In sum, public expenditures for Medicaid have increased, but the burden has fallen more heavily on the federal government than on the states and localities. Moreover, the dollar increase in *state* funds spent on Medicaid was only one-fourth that of the dollar increase in state funds spent for education. Finally, as a proportion of the increase in state moneys spent for all purposes, the Medicaid increase was 15.9 percent of the increase for education and about the same as the increase for highways.

It is of interest, nonetheless, to account for the actual increase in Medicaid expenditures. To do so, we turn to an examination of the right-hand members of the equation.

MEDICAID ELIGIBLES

Since eligibility for Medicaid benefits is, in most instances, predicated on eligibility for public assistance, it is necessary to examine data regarding the eligibles for each of the public assistance categories. Those data are available on a monthly basis because eligiblity is usually reported monthly.[b]

Table 2-2 presents data on the numbers of Medicaid eligibles receiving cash grants under each public assistance category for a winter month and a summer month for the five even-numbered years be-

[a] Apparently, public expenditures for poor people—whether for cash assistance, medical vendor payments, or other services—are viewed differently by the public and treated differently in the press than expenditures for other public purposes. This fact raises at least two sets of questions, both of which are beyond the scope of this book. One concerns how the differences in public attitudes can be accounted for and how, if at all, they can or should be changed. The other concerns whether poor people now get what they need for themselves and for the welfare of the society and, if not, how, in the current context, more can be provided for them. The latter goal might be accomplished, for example, by including their benefits in programs for the entire population through "institutional" or "universal" programs, like national health insurance. See Wilensky and Lebeaux (1958) regarding the distinction between institutional and residual social welfare programs and Titmuss (1965) on universalism in social welfare.

[b] The fact that expenditure data and utilization data are usually calculated on annual bases means that direct comparisons with eligibility figures will not be possible.

Table 2-2. Monthly Numbers of Medicaid Eligibles, February and August, Selected Years, All Reporting States, Grant Cases Only

A. Numbers (in thousands)

	1968 Feb.	1968 Aug.	1970 Feb.	1970 Aug.	1972 Feb.	1972 Aug.	1974 Feb.	1974 Aug.	1976 Feb.	1976 Aug.
Aged	2,060	2,022	2,065	2,054	2,015	2,032	1,883	2,157	2,291	2,203
Blind	82.3	81	80.3	80.2	80.4	81.4	72.6	74.1	75	77
Disabled	654	680	818	899	1,090	1,152	1,281	1,504	1,956	2,007
FDC	5,517	5,705	7,645	8,659	10,809	10,986	10,872	10,764	11,455	11,199
Totals	8,313.3	8,488	10,608.3	11,692.2	13,803.4	14,251.4	14,108.6	14,499.1	15,777	15,486

B. Percent Change

	Feb. 68 Feb. 70	Aug. 68 Aug. 70	Feb. 70 Feb. 72	Aug. 70 Aug. 72	Feb. 72 Feb. 74	Aug. 72 Aug. 74	Feb. 74 Feb. 76	Aug. 74 Aug. 76	Feb. 68 Feb. 76	Aug. 68 Aug. 76
Aged	n.c.	1.6	-2.4	-1.1	-6.6	6.2	21.7	2.1	11.2	9.0
Blind	-2.4	n.c.	n.c.	1.5	-9.7	-9.0	3.3	3.9	-8.9	-4.9
Disabled	25.1	32.2	33.3	28.1	17.5	30.6	52.7	33.4	199.1	195.1
FDC	38.6	51.8	41.4	26.9	n.c.	-2.0	5.4	4.0	107.6	96.3
Totals	27.6	37.7	30.1	21.9	2.2	1.7	11.8	6.8	89.8	82.4

C. Monthly Numbers of Eligibles by Category as Percent of All Eligibles, February and August, Selected Years, Grant Cases Only

	1968 Feb.	1968 Aug.	1970 Feb.	1970 Aug.	1972 Feb.	1972 Aug.	1974 Feb.	1974 Aug.	1976 Feb.	1976 Aug.	Percent Change Feb. 68 Aug. 76	Percent Change Aug. 68 Aug. 76
Aged	24.8	23.8	19.5	17.6	14.6	14.3	13.3	14.9	14.5	14.2	-10.6	-9.6
Blind	<0.01	<0.01	<0.01	<0.01	<0.01	<0.01	<0.01	<0.01	<0.01	<0.01	n.c.	n.c.
Disabled	7.9	8.0	7.7	7.7	7.9	8.1	9.1	10.4	12.4	13.0	5.1	5.0
FDC	66.4	67.2	72.1	74.1	78.3	77.1	77.1	74.2	72.6	72.3	5.9	5.1
Totals	99.1	99.0	99.3	99.4	100.8	99.5	99.5	99.5	99.5	99.5		

Sources: 1968 data: U.S. Bureau of Family Services, *Advance Release of Statistics on Public Assistance*, February and August 1968. 1970 and 1972 data: National Center for Social Statistics, *Public Assistance Statistics*. *NCSS Report A—2*, February and August 1970 and February and August 1972. 1974 and 1976 AFDC data: National Center for Social Statistics, *Public Assistance Statistics*. *NCSS Report A—2*, February and August 1974 and February and August 1976. 1974 and 1976 Aged, Blind, and Disabled data: U.S. Social Security Administration, *Social Security Bulletin*, July 1974, December 1974, and December 1976.

tween 1968 and 1976. Comparisons are made using the same month
from year to year (e.g., February 1968 is compared with February
1970). Examination of those data reveals two points of interest: rates
of growth fluctuated during the period under study, and they varied
considerably from category to category. It can be seen that the numbers of aged eligible for Medicaid showed virtually no change from
February 1968 to February 1970 and a very small (1.6 percent) increase from August 1968 to August 1970. They declined somewhat
during the next three periods but regained the loss between August
1972 and August 1974. Between February 1974 and February 1976
there was a substantial (21.7 percent) gain, but the summer comparisons for those two years showed only a very modest increase. Overall,
there was an increase of about 10 percent from 1968 through 1976.
The large gain may be attributed, in part, to the introduction of the
Supplemental Security Income (SSI) program in January 1974, which
replaced the former state-operated adult categories of public assistance with a new federal program. SSI had the effect of raising the
eligibility levels in some states so that, overnight, more people became eligible for benefits. Additional support for the contribution of
SSI to the growth in eligibles is found in the 6.2 percent increase in
aged eligibles between August 1972 and August 1974. The magnitude of the increase is too large, however, to be explained only by the
introduction of SSI.

In contrast to the experience of the elderly, the numbers of blind
people eligible for Medicaid declined throughout most of the period.
They showed gains in numbers of eligibles only in the last years and
ended the period with fewer eligibles than there were eight years
earlier. The disabled, another adult category, showed substantial bi-
ennial gains throughout the eight-year period, however, almost
tripling the numbers of eligibles between 1968 and 1976.

The largest category, children and adults eligible under the Aid to
Families with Dependent Children (AFDC) programs, also showed
large gains, virtually doubling over the length of the period under
study. After substantial increases over the first four years, however,
AFDC eligibles held steady from 1972 to 1974 and increased modest-
ly thereafter.

As a proportion of the total of eligibles, the aged declined by 10 to
11 percent from 1968 to 1976 because of the increases made by the
disabled and the AFDC eligibles. These trends have implications for
expenditures in that the aged tend to account for relatively more expenditures than children because the aged use both more services
and more expensive services (i.e., hospitals and nursing homes) than
children, and in that services used by the disabled are even more
expensive than those used by the elderly.

These statements about the relative increases and reductions in the proportions of eligibles accounted for by each category must be qualified further by changes in the *numbers* of eligibles. Thus, the 10 percent gain in aged eligibles was accounted for by adding 200,000 elderly to the rolls. The 5 to 9 percent drop for the blind was caused by a loss of only 4,000 to 7,000 people. The disabled tripled by adding about 1 million people to the rolls (six and one-half times the gain in elderly eligibles); and the doubling by the AFDC eligibles was accomplished by the addition of 5.5 to 6 million people (four and one-half times the increase in numbers of disabled eligibles and almost thirty times the growth in numbers of aged eligibles).

Thus, even though more than four and one-half times as many AFDC eligibles joined the rolls as disabled, the fact that care for the disabled costs two to four times as much as care for AFDC recipients means that the expenditure implications of the two very different rates of increase are much closer than the increases in numbers of eligibles. The importance of the changes in numbers of elderly and blind eligibles pales in comparison. This discussion suggests that we need to learn more about the use of services, and we turn to that subject now.

USERS OF SERVICES

The numbers of welfare recipients and medically needy individuals actually using services in the years under study also showed some changes (see Table 2–3). From 1968 through 1976, the numbers of users (that is, the numbers of people for whom medical bills were paid)[c] increased for all categories of eligibility, though at different rates, not only between categories but also from period to period.

For all recipients, the percent increases are substantial, except for the period between 1972 and 1974. For the three largest categories, however, the numbers of users among the elderly increased two to four times more slowly than either the disabled or families with dependent children. Overall, elderly utilizers of services increased by 35 to 60 percent, while the numbers of users among the disabled and families with dependent children more than tripled.

In actual numbers, while the disabled increased at a somewhat faster rate than AFDC families, there were still only about one-

[c] In order to have a complete picture of utilization and of the relationships between eligibility and utilization, data are needed on actual instances of use. Such data are not available on a monthly basis, however, and as a result we are able to consider here only unduplicated counts of users of service. In Chapter 3, annual data on instances of utilization of the most important services are presented.

Table 2-3.   Monthly Numbers of Medicaid Users, All Reporting States February and August, Selected Years

In Thousands

	1968 Feb.	1968 Aug.	1970 Feb.	1970 Aug.	1972 Feb.	1972 Aug.	1974 Feb.	1974 Aug.	1976 Feb.	1976 Aug.	Feb. 68 / Aug. 70	Aug. 68 / Feb. 70	Feb. 70 / Aug. 72	Aug. 70 / Feb. 72	Feb. 72 / Aug. 74	Aug. 72 / Feb. 74	Feb. 74 / Aug. 76	Aug. 74 / Feb. 76	Feb. 68 / Feb. 76	Aug. 68 / Aug. 76
											Percent Change									
All Recipients																				
Aged	1,254	1,389	1,453	1,577	1,927	1,855	1,776	1,800	2,006	1,984	15.9	13.5	32.6	17.6	−7.8	−3.0	13.0	10.2	60.0	36.5
Blind	33	36	37	44	50	47	47	46	45	43	12.1	22.2	35.1	6.8	−6.0	−2.1	−4.3	−6.5	36.4	19.4
Disabled	360	425	550	629	837	893	936	973	1,239	1,289	52.8	48.0	52.2	42.0	11.8	9.0	32.4	32.5	244.2	203.3
FDC	1,545	1,703	2,757	2,912	3,708	3,703	3,867	3,882	4,840	4,645	63.6	71.0	46.7	27.2	4.3	4.8	25.2	19.7	213.3	172.8
Totals[a]	3,749	4,090	4,908	5,503	7,014	6,907	7,292	7,212	8,729	8,526	30.9	34.5	42.9	25.5	4.0	4.4	19.7	18.2	132.8	108.5
Grant Cases Only																				
Aged	761	818	902	995	1,237	1,201	1,030	1,093	1,243	1,218	18.5	21.6	37.1	20.7	−167	−9.0	20.7	11.4	63.3	48.9
Blind	30	32	33	38	45	42	41	40	37	36	11.0	18.4	35.1	10.5	−9.6	−5.2	−9.8	−16.2	23.3	12.5
Disabled	286	331	434	502	672	693	735	767	947	998	51.7	51.7	54.8	38.0	9.4	10.7	28.8	30.1	231.1	201.5
FDC	1,175	1,335	2,061	2,377	3,319	3,280	3,437	3,473	4,370	4,204	75.4	78.1	61.0	38.0	3.6	5.9	27.1	21.0	271.9	214.9
Totals	2,328	2,630	3,612	4,086	5,473	5,216	5,243	5,373	6,597	6,456	52.3	119.0	53.7	33.3	−0.6	3.0	25.8	20.2	183.4	154.5
Nongrant Cases																				
Aged	494	571	553	581	688	654	746	706	743	745	11.9	1.8	24.4	12.6	8.4	8.0	<0.01	5.5	50.4	30.5
Blind	3	3	4	6	5	5	6	6	8	7	33.3	100.0	25.0	−167	20.0	20.0	33.3	16.7	166.7	133.3
Disabled	75	94	115	127	163	200	201	206	282	281	53.3	35.1	41.7	57.5	23.3	3.0	40.3	36.4	276.0	198.9
FDC	371	369	466	536	389	422	430	409	438	412	25.6	45.3	−16.5	−213	10.5	−3.1	1.9	n.c.	18.1	11.7
Totals[a]	1,420	1,460	1,296	1,418	1,539	1,690	2,050	1,840	2,066	2,006	−8.7	−2.9	18.8	19.2	33.2	8.9	<0.01	9.0	45.5	37.4

Sources: NCSS, B-1 Reports.

[a]Totals include, in some cases, recipients not apportioned to grant and nongrant status as well as recipients in nonfederally aided categories.

fourth the number of disabled users of services as AFDC users. Moreover, although gains in the elderly category were relatively modest in percentage terms, they were much closer to the disabled in actual numbers of users. Finally, the increase in numbers of AFDC families using services was three to four times the increase in users among the disabled.

Users who also received cash grants were more than three times as numerous as the medically needy, but again there are differences among categories. Rates of increase generally paralleled the overall increases with two exceptions. In the small category of blind people, the medically needy increased at a rate seven to ten times as fast as grant recipients. In the more significant AFDC category, the number of medically needy users increased hardly at all over the entire eight-year period and, moreover, the entire gain was accounted for in the first two years of the study period. Since the rates of expenditure for medically needy users tend to be higher than those for public assistance recipients, the general tendency should be to increase costs even more than is apparent from the substantial increases in numbers of eligibles and users of services. That issue will be treated below.

EXPENDITURES BY CATEGORY

Now that it has been noted that the numbers of eligibles and the numbers of users of services have been increasing in all eligibility categories, we can shed additional light on the growth in expenditures by examining them, too, by category of eligibility.

Overall, monthly expenditures for all recipients almost quadrupled between 1968 and 1976, amounting to approximately $1.25 billion a month by the end of the period (see Table 2–4). The largest percentage gains were recorded by the disabled, followed by families with dependent children. Expenditures for the disabled increased by four and one-half to five and one-half times during the eight years, while outlays for families with dependent children grew by three and one-half to more than four times. Expenditures for care received by the elderly tripled.

These relative proportional gains, however, belie the fact that the elderly accounted for more dollars spent than any other group although their relatively lower rate of increase meant that the gap with other groups narrowed during the period. The difference was attributable to the much heavier use of the program by the medically needy elderly than by the medically needy in any other category. Among nongrant cases, the elderly accounted for more than two and one-half times the expenditures accounted for by the disabled, who

Table 2–4.   Monthly Payments for Medical Services by Basis of Recipient Eligibility, All Reporting States, 1968–1976

thousands of dollars

	1968		1970		1972		1974		1976	
	Feb.	*Aug.*	*Feb.*	*Aug.*	*Feb.*	*Aug.*	*Feb.*	*Aug.*	*Feb.*	*Aug.*
All Recipients										
Aged	123,899	149,271	158,024	172,088	240,775	272,162	296,197	337,930	410,836	443,444
Blind	2,455	2,618	2,726	3,812	5,365	4,741	6,449	6,241	7,012	7,907
Disabled	43,744	56,262	82,559	88,084	138,980	165,740	177,297	194,344	280,895	320,158
FDC	68,141	84,393	127,676	144,267	199,639	225,259	248,358	278,751	352,358	388,780
Other	47,333	40,425	31,797	27,863	43,829	47,084	50,337	52,406	67,114	78,656
Totals	281,850[a]	335,973	402,784	436,105	628,587	714,986	786,208	869,646	1,118,215	1,238,945
Grant Cases Only										
Aged	42,155	51,536	43,669	66,634	71,439	80,259	79,918	91,848	118,530	126,581
Blind	1,874	2,014	2,218	3,018	3,986	3,599	4,264	4,090	4,327	5,216
Disabled	27,988	36,275	53,764	56,032	89,976	105,517	113,917	117,142	172,888	202,069
FDC	50,347	63,995	98,293	115,862	169,780	193,091	210,718	235,631	304,828	333,440
Other	6,594	8,269	11,541	9,891	17,090	—[b]	—	—	—	—
Totals	128,958[a]	165,080	219,480	251,433	352,272	382,465	408,817	448,711	600,573	667,306
Nongrant Cases										
Aged	81,744	97,735	104,358	105,450	165,299	191,903	216,279	246,082	288,695	313,401
Blind	579	605	509	795	1,377	1,142	2,186	2,124	2,629	2,671
Disabled	15,753	19,993	28,792	32,057	48,076	60,223	63,380	77,202	105,293	115,421
FDC	17,793	20,400	29,386	28,405	29,858	32,169	37,640	43,121	45,459	53,209
Other	35,738	32,158	20,254	17,970	26,732	—	—	—	—	—
Totals	152,890[a]	170,889	183,300	184,674	271,342	332,520	377,392	420,935	508,708	562,970

Percent Change

	Feb. 68 *Feb. 70*	*Aug. 68* *Aug. 70*	*Feb. 70* *Feb. 72*	*Aug. 70* *Aug. 72*	*Feb. 72* *Feb. 74*	*Aug. 72* *Aug. 74*	*Feb. 74* *Feb. 76*	*Aug. 74* *Aug. 76*	*Feb. 68* *Feb. 76*	*Aug. 68* *Aug. 76*
All Recipients										
Aged	27.5	15.3	52.4	58.2	23.0	24.2	38.7	31.2	231.6	197.1
Blind	11.0	45.6	96.8	24.4	20.2	31.1	47.9	26.7	185.6	202.0
Disabled	88.7	56.6	68.3	88.2	27.6	17.3	58.4	64.7	542.1	469.0
FDC	87.4	70.9	56.4	56.1	24.4	23.7	41.9	39.5	417.1	360.7
Other	-24.9	-31.1	37.8	69.0	14.8	11.3	33.3	50.1	58.5	94.6
Totals	42.9	29.8	56.1	63.9	25.1	21.6	42.2	42.5	296.7	268.8
Grant Cases Only										
Aged	3.6	29.3	63.6	20.4	11.9	14.4	48.3	37.8	181.2	145.6
Blind	18.4	49.9	79.7	19.3	7.0	13.6	1.5	27.5	130.9	159.0
Disabled	92.1	54.5	67.4	88.3	26.6	11.0	51.8	72.5	517.7	457.0
FDC	95.2	81.0	72.7	66.7	24.1	22.0	44.7	41.5	505.5	421.0
Other	75.0	19.6	48.1	—	—	—	—	—	—	—
Totals	70.2	52.3	45.6	52.1	16.1	17.3	46.9	48.7	365.7	304.2
Nongrant Cases										
Aged	27.7	7.9	58.4	82.0	30.8	28.2	33.5	27.4	253.2	220.7
Blind	-12.1	31.4	170.5	43.6	58.8	86.0	20.3	25.8	354.1	341.5
Disabled	82.8	60.3	67.0	87.9	31.8	28.2	66.1	49.5	568.4	477.3
FDC	65.2	39.2	1.6	13.2	26.1	34.0	20.8	23.4	155.5	160.8
Other	-43.3	-44.1	32.0	—	—	—	—	—	—	—
Totals	19.9	8.1	48.0	80.1	39.1	26.6	34.8	33.7	232.7	229.4

Source: NCSS, B-1 Reports

[a]Totals include small amounts not distributed by eligibility.

[b]Data not available after Feb. 1972.

Table 2-5. Monthly Number of Grant Recipient Users of Medicaid Services as Percent of All Users, Selected Years

	1968		1970		1972		1974		1976	
	Feb.	Aug.	Feb.	Aug.	Feb.	Aug.	Feb.	Aug.	Feb.	Aug.
Aged	60.7	58.9	62.1	63.1	64.2	64.7	58.0	60.7	62.0	61.4
Blind	90.9	88.9	89.2	86.4	90.0	89.4	87.2	87.0	82.2	83.7
Disabled	79.4	77.9	78.9	79.8	80.3	77.6	78.5	78.8	76.4	77.4
FDC	76.1	78.4	81.6	81.6	89.5	88.6	88.9	89.5	90.3	90.5
Totals	62.1	64.3	73.6	74.3	78.0	75.5	71.9	74.5	75.6	75.7

Monthly Medicaid Payments for Grant Recipients as Precent of Payments for All Recipients

	1968		1970		1972		1974		1976	
	Feb.	Aug.	Feb.	Aug.	Feb.	Aug.	Feb.	Aug.	Feb.	Aug.
Aged	34.0	34.5	27.6	38.7	29.7	29.5	27.0	27.2	28.9	28.5
Blind	76.3	76.9	81.4	79.2	74.3	75.9	67.7	65.8	61.7	66.0
Disabled	64.0	64.5	65.1	63.6	64.7	63.7	64.3	60.3	61.5	63.1
FDC	73.9	75.8	77.0	80.3	85.0	85.7	84.8	84.5	86.5	85.8
Totals	45.8	49.1	54.5	57.7	56.0	53.5	52.0	51.6	53.7	53.9

Source: Tables 2–3 and 2–4.

represented the next largest category (Tables 2–4 and 2–5). Also, almost 40 percent of elderly recipients were nongrant recipients and more than 70 percent of the money spent on the elderly went for nongrant recipients (Table 2–5). These figures contrast sharply with those in the other categories. In no other group do the medically needy represent more than 25 percent of users of service or account for more than 40 percent of funds. The impact of the medically needy program is examined more fully in Chapter 5.

EXPENDITURES PER PERSON

The foregoing array of numbers leaves the general impression of continual growth in all eligibility categories, whether we are measuring the numbers of eligibles, the numbers of users of services, or the amount of money spent. The totals are dazzling for their sheer magnitude. We need to reduce them to understandable levels. In Table 2–6, the gross amounts are reduced to expenditures for an average individual who is eligible for the program and for an average individual who uses services. Again, substantial differences can be observed between eligiblity categories.

Looking first at eligibles, while more people qualified for Medicaid benefits under the AFDC program, less is spent on each eligible person under that category than in any other. And although the amount spent per AFDC eligible in 1976 was almost triple the amount spent in 1968, the value of the services each received then was still the lowest of any category. Similarly, the largest amount was spent on the average disabled eligible at the beginning of the period and at the end. An eligible person in the third major category, the elderly, was second lowest in three of the four months for which data are presented. The last finding is somewhat surprising until we remember that the medically needy, who are unrepresented in these figures, account for the majority of expenditures for the elderly. Finally, when the four eligibility categories are compared for the percentage change in amount spent per eligible, the disabled are the only category with a rate of increase below that for the entire group. Expenditures per eligible in the other categories grew by two and one-half to three times, with the largest rate of increase found among the families with dependent children.

When we turn to those who have actually used services, it is possible to examine not only totals, but also figures for the medically needy as well as for the grant recipients in each category. Again, overall, the rankings among the four categories remained stable, with individuals under the AFDC category accounting for the lowest per capita expenditures and the disabled accounting for the highest.

Table 2-6 Monthly Medicaid Expenditures per Eligible and per User, 1968 and 1976

	A. Monthly Amount Spent per Eligible (dollars)				B. Monthly Amount Spent per User (dollars)				C. Percent Change in Amount Spent per User	
	Feb. 68	Feb. 76	Aug. 68	Aug. 76	Feb. 68	Feb. 76	Aug. 68	Aug. 76	Feb. 68 Feb. 76	Aug. 68 Aug. 76
Grant Cases										
Aged	20.46	51.74	25.49	57.46	55.39	95.36	63.00	103.93	72.2	65.0
Blind	22.85	57.69	24.86	67.74	62.47	116.95	62.94	144.89	87.2	130.2
Disabled	42.80	88.39	53.35	100.68	97.86	182.56	109.59	202.47	86.6	84.8
FDC	9.13	26.61	11.22	29.77	42.85	69.75	47.94	79.31	62.8	65.4
Totals	15.51	38.07	19.45	43.09	55.39	91.04	62.77	103.36	64.4	64.7
Nongrant Cases										
Aged					165.47	388.55	171.16	420.67	134.8	145.7
Blind					193.00	328.63	201.67	381.57	70.3	89.2
Disabled					210.04	373.38	212.69	410.75	77.8	93.1
FDC					47.96	103.79	55.28	129.15	116.4	133.6
Totals					107.67	246.23	117.05	280.64	128.7	139.8
All Cases										
Aged					98.80	204.80	107.47	223.51	107.3	108.0
Blind					74.39	155.82	72.72	183.88	109.5	152.9
Disabled					121.51	226.71	132.38	248.38	86.6	87.6
FDC					44.10	72.80	49.56	83.70	65.1	68.9
Totals					75.18	128.10	82.14	145.31	70.4	76.9

D. Percent Change in Amount Spent per Eligible, Grant Cases

	Feb. 68 Feb. 76	Aug. 68 Aug. 76
Aged	152.9	125.4
Blind	152.5	172.5
Disabled	106.5	88.7
FDC	191.5	165.3
Total	145.5	121.5

E. Percent Change in Amount Spent per Nongrant Recipient User Minus Percent Change in Amount Spent per Grant Recipient User

	Feb. 68 Feb. 76	Aug. 68 Aug. 76
Aged	62.6	80.7
Blind	-16.9	-41.0
Disabled	-8.8	8.3
FDC	53.6	68.2
Total	64.3	75.1

While the elderly individual was third among users, as among eligibles, in this case he or she was much closer to the costly disabled individual than to the relatively inexpensive AFDC service user. That shift is accounted for by the fact that, among nongrant recipients, the elderly individual accounted for more than $420 per user, more than any other category. The disabled were second and the blind were third, while the average AFDC nongrant recipient trailed a distant fourth. The fact that, in all cases, the average medically needy user of services accounted for more money than the average grant recipient is understandable when it is recognized that he or she was likely to seek benefits under the program only when ill with a relatively serious condition; that is, when the expenses for medical care became a more-than-usual burden. The public assistance recipient, in contrast, used services for less severe conditions as well as for serious ones. He was eligible for benefits as long as he received public assistance, not just when he became ill. Even the rate of increase for the medically needy was in most cases higher than that for grant recipients (Table 2–6).

The rates of change in per capita expenditures for users of service over the eight-year period are relatively modest compared to changes in the amount spent per eligible person. Among grant recipients, the average amount spent per user of service increased by only about 65 percent for all categories considered together. Expenditures for the average disabled individual using services grew by another 20 percent, and those for the average blind user grew even more. (Since the number of blind eligibles is so small, however, the impact of this higher rate of growth is also small.)

Increases for the medically needy were higher than those for grant recipients, especially for the elderly and AFDC categories. Overall, the percent change for all categories was approximately 75 percent. The blind and elderly individuals received services worth approximately one-third more than that.

SUMMARY AND CONCLUSIONS

Table 2–7 summarizes the trend data presented in Tables 2–2 through 2–6 and allows us to draw tentative conclusions about the reasons for increasing Medicaid expenditures. Columns A, B, and C record the percent change observed in previous tables for the monthly number of eligibles, the monthly number of recipients of services, and monthly expenditures. The final two columns compare them.

It can be seen that while the number of eligibles increased in all but the small category of blind people, the numbers of users of services increased by substantially larger amounts. Thus, in the large

Table 2-7.   Percent Change, 1968–1976, Selected Measures

	A. Monthly Eligibles Grant Cases		B. Monthly Recipients Grant Cases		C. Monthly Expenditures Grant Cases		D. Percent Change in Recipients Minus Eligibles		E. Percent Change in Expenditures Minus Percent Change in Recipients	
	Feb. 68–76	Aug. 68–76	Feb. 68–76	Aug. 68–76	Feb. 68–76	Aug. 68–76	Feb. 68–76	Aug. 68–76	Feb. 68–76	Aug. 68–76
Aged	11.2	9.0	63.3	48.9	181.2	145.6	52.1	39.9	117.9	96.7
Blind	-8.9	-4.9	23.3	12.5	130.9	159.0	32.2	17.4	107.6	146.5
Disabled	199.1	195.1	231.1	201.5	517.7	457.0	32.0	6.4	286.6	255.5
FDC	107.6	96.3	271.9	214.9	505.5	421.0	164.3	118.6	233.6	206.1
Totals	89.8	82.4	183.4	154.5	365.7	304.2	93.6	72.1	182.3	149.7
Non Grant Cases										
Aged			50.4	30.5	253.2	220.7			202.8	190.2
Blind			166.7	133.3	354.1	341.5			187.4	208.2
Disabled			276.0	198.9	568.4	477.3			292.4	278.4
FDC			18.1	11.7	155.5	160.8			137.4	149.1
Totals			45.5	37.4	232.7	229.4			187.2	192.0
All Cases										
Aged			60.0	36.5	231.6	197.1			171.6	160.6
Blind			36.4	19.4	185.6	202.0			149.2	182.6
Disabled			244.2	203.3	542.1	469.0			297.9	265.7
FDC			213.3	172.8	417.1	360.7			203.8	187.9
Totals			132.8	108.5	296.7	268.8			163.9	160.3

AFDC category, while the number of eligibles doubled, the number of users of services more than tripled. In the other categories, the differences were smaller, but not insubstantial.

The most dramatic differences, however, were registered in the expenditure columns themselves. There it can be seen that expenditures grew two and one-half to four times faster than the number of recipients of service, which, we saw, grew almost twice as fast as the number of eligibles. The figures are higher for the medically needy than for grant recipients.

Although the data show that the number of eligibles can still explain some of the growth in Medicaid expenditures, it is no longer the dominant factor. Moreover, Table 2–7 shows that expenditures have been increasing even faster than users of services. On the basis of these data we are not yet able to sort out the relative contribution of price and the amount of services used to explain that residual, however. For the time being, therefore, we must be content with the conclusion that much of the increase in expenditures is left unexplained by the growth in numbers of eligibles and numbers of users of services. At the end of the next chapter, following a discussion of the utilization of services, I will have more to say about that question.

3

Utilization of Services

Medicaid expenditures are the result of the number of people using services, the rate of service use, and the price of those services. As indicated in Chapter 2, much of the growth in expenditures in the program can be explained by increases in the numbers of eligibles and, even more importantly, by gains in the numbers of users of services. But much is left unexplained. More must be learned about the utilization of services by those who find a need for medical care and about the price of that care. The discussion in this chapter will concentrate on utilization. First, a general introduction to the question of what utilization means will be presented. Then data from Medicaid programs will be introduced in an attempt to add to the conclusions drawn in Chapter 2, principally through a discussion of utilization rates. Finally, expenditures will be linked to utilization rates in a way that allows some attention to the contribution of the price of services to aggregate expenditures.

DEFINITION AND MEASUREMENT

Medicaid program analysts are accustomed to considering the utilization of services in aggregate terms. It is worth remembering, however, that those aggregates consist of individual decisions made by millions of people. Moreover, an individual's decision to utilize a particular medical service is the result of a complex of interrelated factors whose relative importance varies with the nature of the individual's condition and the type of service. At any time, every person can be located on a continuum from absolute health to critical illness, and the amount of discretion a person has in the selection of services varies with his or her position on that continuum. For example, a person who has a heart attack is likely to have less discretion and a more limited range of medical care options to choose from than a person who has a cold and for whom even no care is a viable option. The relationship between health status and the discretion available to an individual is shown graphically in Figure 3–1.

Discretion in Seeking Medical Services	Very Great	Great	Consid- erable	None	
Health Status	Healthy	"Worried Well"	"Not Feeling Well"	Acutely Ill	Critically Ill

Figure 3–1. Parallel Continua Showing Relationship between Health Status and Amount of Discretion Available to Individual Regarding the Use of Medical Services

A number of reseachers have developed models that provide insights into consumer discretion in the use of medical services (see, for example, Andersen, 1968; Andersen and Newman, 1973; and Hershey, Luft, and Gianaris, 1975). Typically, they include characteristics of the individual decisionmaker (e.g., age, sex, race, income, attitudes, health status) and characteristics of the system in which the care is to be sought (e.g., availability of practitioners and facilities, organizational modes, financing mechanisms).

Numerous empirical studies have demonstrated that these factors do indeed affect the use of medical services, and some have attempted to identify the relative importance of each (see Andersen, Kravits, and Anderson, 1975, for a recent study; Aday and Eichhorn, 1973, provide an extensive bibliography). The evidence from these studies indicates that the patient occupies the key role at the point of deciding whether to seek care at all (i.e., enter the system) and that, beyond that point, the physician is more influential (Foster, 1977). The point, for our purposes, is that utilization is the result of many factors, only one of which is the patient's ability to pay.

Optimal utilization might be defined as the congruence of need and utilization. At any one time in any place the patterns for particular services may or may not reflect optimal responses to some objective measure of physical need. Of course, in our complex world the presence of a measurable physical ailment may not be the only legitimate reason for the use of services. The decision to use a particular service—or indeed the decision to seek medical care at all—includes other important considerations that must be acknowledged.

Since Medicaid expenditures are, most directly, the result of the utilization of medical services, it is worth considering briefly some of the determinants of utilization and, particularly, the relationship of demand to the need for care.[a] In simple terms, *demand* is the level of services a person wants, modified by some presumed calculation of whether that person wants or is able to pay the going price for it. As Boulding points out (1973: 3, 17), the concept of demand rests on the notion of consumer sovereignty as a preferred value. What the consumer buys is what he or she *should* buy because the purchase decision encompasses, at least in theory, a weighing of the presumed benefits of the service and the anticipated costs. Thus, some may be led to equate demand with the need for care or at least to say that, on these grounds, it is sufficient to examine only demand because the sovereign consumer has already considered the need for services in deciding to act or not. But this view must be qualified by several factors including, among others, consumer ignorance, income, and the supply of services.

One difficulty that arises when this notion is applied to the medical arena is that the seller, the professional provider of care, knows a good deal more about the services and their presumed effects on the consumer's condition than does the consumer. Moreover, the greater the educational and cultural distance between the provider and the patient—as for example in the case of most Medicaid patients—the more likely is this pattern to occur. It is important because ignorance may lead people to miscalculate their true need or misjudge its importance and thus to demand services that are not medically good for them or to overlook services that are essential. Thus demand is not a satisfactory reflection of the need for medical services because consumers are usually unable to evaluate the alternatives available to them—if indeed they know what they are—because they do not have sufficient knowledge of their likely outcomes.

Another difficulty in equating need and demand for medical services is that some who would like to buy services are unable to do so because they do not have enough money. Most societies, including our own, have standards that call for the provision of a "social minimum" (Boulding, 1973: 18) for those who are not able to obtain it legitimately on their own, and medical care is an area in which such

---

[a] For more complete discussions of the determinants of utilization, the reader is referred to the sources cited.

provisions are generally made. Title XIX of the Social Security Act, the Medicaid title, is one expression of that view.

Although Medicaid and other public programs have enhanced the capacity of some groups of people to buy medical care, gaps remain. While patterns of use for different income groups have been narrowing, the benefits of these programs are not distributed equally among all the poor (see Bice, Eichhorn, and Fox, 1972; Davis and Reynolds, 1976; Davis and Schoen, 1978). Moreover, using different measures of the need for services, several authors have found that poor people are still probably underusers of medical services (Aday, 1976; Kravits and Schneider, 1975; Davis and Reynolds, 1976).

Finally, need and demand cannot be equated because, to some extent, the presence of a supply of services *creates* the demand for them. Thus, as Roemer has shown, rates of hospitalization and length of stay increase with the supply of hospital beds in a community (Roemer, 1961). The use of certain kinds of physicians' services, too, apparently increases as the supply of specialists increases (Stevens, 1971; Bunker, 1970; Vayda, 1973). This is not to say that the increased utilization is medically inappropriate, but only to note that utilization is influenced by the available supply of services. Understanding that utilization rates are influenced by the supply of services is important, in part because, although they presumably have, through the program, the ability to pay for services, Medicaid patients often reside in areas with limited medical resources.

It is also important to understand more about the role of the physician, who usually stands as the point of first contact to the medical care system when an individual decides to seek services. Robert Evans, an economist, points out that a physician, who is the gatekeeper to many medical services, typically performs two roles at the same time. In one, he acts as "the agent of the patient," diagnosing and treating the condition for which he is consulted. In the other, "he is a supplier of a particular class of services whose income and work satisfaction are related to the volume of services he supplies and the price he receives for them" (Evans, 1974: 162–3).

George Monsma, another economist, writes that financial considerations affect medical decisions and in some cases are a "decisive factor" in the recommendation of treatment. He concludes, with appropriate academic restraint, that "the effect of the monetary factor is not so weak as always to be insignificant" (Monsma, 1970: 145–46).

Bunker's research, too, supports this view (Bunker, 1979; see also Vayda, 1973; Wennberg and Gittelsohn, 1973). He found surgeon/population ratios in the United States twice as large as in England and Wales and rates of surgery two or more times as great

(1970: 136). He concluded that the higher rates for many surgical procedures in the United States are less likely to be attributable to such large differences in the incidence of the conditions that the procedures are intended to correct than to nonmedical factors that encourage the training of more surgeons who, naturally, perform more surgery. Among these are the organization, structure, and financing of medical care, and differences in the styles of medical practice in the two countries.

It is not necessary to accept a view of physicians as single-minded, income-maximizing, economic rationalists to believe that they exercise considerable influence on the demand for their services. Their recommendations to patients and, therefore, their influence on the demand for services may well arise from factors other than economic self-interest. It may be that they have confidence in the services they have to offer, even in the absence of controlled evidence to support the choice of those services over others or over none. And it may be that they, like others, feel a compulsion to "do something" when confronted with a problem. But, whatever their motives, it is clear that physicians do exercise "direct, nonprice influence" on the patient's demand for services (Evans, 1974: 162) and that the effect of their behavior is to increase demand and hence their incomes.

The role of the physician-gatekeeper is central to an understanding of the utilization of medical services. For the Medicaid analyst or policymaker, the question is how to influence the doctor to act so that Medicaid patients receive services which approximate their need and so that the cost implications of his actions are a factor in his decision as well. The answer, I believe, lies in appreciation of his dual position as a professional trained to exercise judgment when his knowledge, though greater than the patient's, is still imperfect; and as a person whose livelihood depends on the provision of services. The proposals made in Chapter 8 are based, in part, on this recognition.

This very brief introduction to the utilization literature, while not doing justice to the complexity of the subject, shows that consumer demand for medical services is influenced by consumer ignorance, the ability to pay for care, the local supply of services, and the physician's role as gatekeeper to the medical care system. These factors, as well as others (see, for example, Andersen and Newman 1973), moderate the impact of the patient's need on the decision to utilize services. They justify the view that utilization figures are not accurate representations of the need for services by Medicaid patients and that some of the discrepancy may be on the side of overutilization. Thus, when program costs are thought to be too high, attempting to reduce expenditures by reducing utilization is an appropriate strategy to be considered. But, if it is to succeed, such a strategy must be based on a sufficient understanding of the dynamics of the medical care system which produce utilization.

Medicaid was designed to remove financial incapacity as a barrier to the utilization of medical services, and, to the extent it was successful in doing so, utilization should have increased for Medicaid eligibles. As we saw in the last chapter, that is, in fact, the case.

In the pages that follow, annual data from Medicaid programs are presented by eligibility category and by type of service used. These data will make possible a better explanation of the growth in Medicaid utilization and Medicaid expenditures.

UTILIZATION OF SERVICES UNDER MEDICAID

By Eligibility

Between 1968 and 1976, the number of recipients of medical services under Medicaid doubled from 12.2 million to 24.7 million (Table 3–1).[b] There were substantial gains in the number of recipients in each category of eligibility, but the greatest proportional gain by far was among the disabled. They more than tripled their numbers from 840,000 to 2.7 million, although the disabled still accounted for more than 1 million fewer recipients than the elderly.

The number of elderly recipients increased by less than 40 percent, probably because large increases in the number of the elderly poor receiving medical assistance had occurred under the Kerr-Mills Act, passed five years before Medicaid became effective, and because Medicare, which covers more than 90 percent of the elderly, poor and nonpoor alike, took care of much of the need of older Americans for acute care and kept many from becoming poor enough to qualify for Medicaid.

The largest categories were individuals eligible as members of families with dependent children. Further, while there were 2.5 children for every AFDC adult using services in 1968, by 1976 that number had fallen to two children for each adult because AFDC adults increased at a higher rate than children.

The proportion of users accounted for by each eligibility category has been remarkably constant; the fluctuations that can be observed are relatively small (Table 3–2). The largest and steadiest tendency has been for the proportion represented by the elderly to decline, reflecting primarily the large increases in the numbers of AFDC adults and the disabled.

[b] We began with 1968 since it is the first year after the implementation of Medicaid for which utilization data are available.

Table 3-1. Annual Recipients of Medicaid Services, 1968–1976
(in thousands)

	1968	1969	CY[c] 1970	FY[c] 1971[a]	1972	1973	1974	1975	1976	Percent Income 1972–1976	Percent Income 1968–1976
A. By Basis of Eligibility											
Aged	2,747	2,870	3,529	3,600	3,417	3,549	3,805	3,699	3,808	11.4	38.6
Blind	64	98	110	123	109	102	136	107	98	−10.1	53.1
Disabled	842	1,033	1,432	1,500	1,673	1,843	2,280	2,308	2,664	59.2	216.4
AFDC adults	2,228	3,132	3,392	4,700	3,196	4,146	4,511	4,662	5,238	63.9	135.1
AFDC children	5,574	6,517	7,242	8,300	8,177	8,826	9,730	9,776	10,645	30.2	91.0
Totals	12,194	14,612	16,419	19,323	18,312	19,999	22,009	22,413	24,666	34.7	102.3
B. By Type of Service Used											
Gen. hosp.	1,884	2,222	2,542		2,935	3,308	3,359	3,485	3,614	23.1	91.8
SNF[a]	541	578	591		562	689	676	623	636	13.2	17.6
ICF[a]	67	—	—		—	470	644	712	792	68.5[b]	1,082.1
Physicians	7,596	9,077	10,417	not	12,699	13,482	15,286	15,451	15,923	25.4	109.6
Outpatient hosp.	2,626	3,281	4,131	available	5,487	5,296	5,699	6,071	7,448	35.7	183.6
Clinic	101	542	595		521	1,981	2,147	2,431	2,255	332.8	2,132.7
Lab & X-ray	910	1,365	1,517		3,628	4,065	4,171	4,392	4,995	37.7	448.9
Prescribed drugs	6,820	8,534	9,859		11,522	12,277	14,543	14,070	15,040	30.5	120.5
All	12,194	14,612	16,419		18,312	19,999	22,009	22,413	24,666	34.7	102.3
All Nursing Homes[a]	608	578	591		562	1,159	1,320	1,335	1,428	154.1	134.9

Source: National Center for Social Statistics (later, Health Care Financing Administration), Report B-4 for 1968–1976, except Report B-5 for 1971. Totals include estimates for nonreporting states.

[a] All Nursing Homes = skilled nursing facilities and intermediate care facilities.

[b] Percent increase for ICF calculated for 1973–1976.

[c] CY = Calendar year (1968–1970)

  FY = Fiscal year (1971–1976)

Table 3-2   Recipients By Category as a Proportion of All Recipients

(In percent)

A. By Basis of Eligibility

	1968	1969	1970	1971	1972	1973	1974	1975	1976	Change 1972–1976	1968–1976
Aged	22.5	19.6	21.5	18.6	18.7	17.7	17.3	16.5	15.4	−3.3	−7.1
Blind	0.5	0.7	0.7	0.6	0.6	0.5	0.6	0.5	0.4	−0.2	−0.1
Disabled	6.9	7.1	8.7	7.8	9.1	9.2	10.4	10.3	10.8	1.7	3.9
AFDC adults	19.3	21.4	20.7	24.3	17.5	20.7	20.5	20.8	21.2	3.7	2.9
AFDC children	45.7	44.6	44.1	43.0	44.7	44.1	44.2	43.6	43.2	−1.5	−2.5
Total	93.9	93.4	95.7	94.3	90.6	92.2	93.0	91.7	91.0	0.4	−2.9

B. By Type of Service Used

	1968	1969	1970	1971	1972	1973	1974	1975	1976	Change 1972–1976	1968–1976
Gen. hosp.	15.5	15.2	15.5	not avail-able	16.0	16.5	15.3	15.5	14.7	−1.3	−0.8
SNF	4.4	4.0	3.6		3.1	3.4	3.1	2.8	2.6	−0.5	−1.8
ICF	0.5	—	—		—	2.4	2.9	3.2	3.2	0.8	+3.2
Physicians	62.3	62.1	63.4		69.3	67.4	69.5	68.9	64.6	−4.7	+2.3
Outpatient hosp.	21.5	22.5	25.2		30.0	26.5	25.9	27.1	30.2	0.2	8.7
Clinic	0.8	3.7	3.6		2.8	9.9	9.8	10.8	9.1	6.3	9.1
Lab & X-ray	7.5	9.3	9.2		19.8	20.3	19.0	19.6	20.3	0.5	12.8
Prescribed drugs	55.9	58.4	60.0		62.9	61.4	66.1	62.8	61.0	−1.9	5.1

Source: National Center for Social Statistics (later, Health Care Financing Administration), Report B-4 for 1968–1976, except Report B-5 for 1971. Totals include estimates for nonreporting states.

aPercent increase for ICF calculated for 1973–1976

By Type of Service

The numbers of persons using the various services increased dramatically. In fact, for all but one category (users of hospital services) the 1976 figures more than doubled those for 1968 (see Table 3–1). The numbers of people using physician services grew by 110 percent and those using prescribed drugs by 120 percent. Users of laboratory and X-ray services increased by almost 450 percent, and users of clinic services by more than 2,100 percent (although they still represented only 9 percent of all recipients).

The users of nursing home services increased by 135 percent, which is accounted for primarily by the coverage in 1973 of care given in intermediate care facilities (IFC). Users of skilled nursing facilities (SNF), which are covered in part by Medicare for both the elderly and the disabled, grew in numbers by only 18 percent. Together, ICF and SNF users represent a substantial part of the large chronic care component of Medicaid; Medicare covers the first twenty days of care in an SNF and does not cover ICF services at all.

The number of recipients using ambulatory medical services grew by more than 15 million during this period. Of this growth, 46 percent was accounted for by hospital outpatient departments (including emergency departments) and free-standing clinics and 54 percent by physicians. Proportionally, outpatient departments and clinics almost doubled their share of users of services, from 22.3 percent in 1968 to 39.3 percent in 1976. Moreover, at the same time that the proportion of recipients using those services increased so dramatically, the percentage using physicians also increased somewhat.

Users of physicians' services, as a proportion of users of all services, fluctuated within a relatively narrow range showing only a 2.3 percent larger share in 1976 (Table 3–2). But if these users are added to users of hospital outpatient services and clinic services, the proportion of people receiving ambulatory care from all sources grew by almost 20 percent. It is not possible to determine precisely what proportion of physician service users were ambulatory, however, since approximately 16 percent of physician visits occurred with hospital inpatients. Undoubtedly, most of those patients also saw physicians in offices, clinics, or outpatient departments.

The extent to which clinic use represents a substitution of one site of care for another cannot be determined with the available data. It is not clear, for example, how many users of private physicians were also users, at other times, of hospital emergency rooms (ER) and outpatient departments or of free-standing clinics; but it is likely that at least some people used both sources of ambulatory care since the proportion seeing a physician changed relatively little while the proportion using the other sources increased markedly. It is also not clear how much of that use reflected changes in the regular source of care and how much represented the habitual use of multiple sources. (Some people, for example, use ERs when their regular physician is unavailable. Such people would show up as users of both sources.)

Only part of the utilization picture is provided by the number of users of each service. It is also necessary to consider the rates of use by each recipient. The question to ask is how much has utilization by individual recipients of service changed?

By Individual Rates

Data on the *numbers of users* of services are available since 1968, but figures for *use* of the most heavily utilized services have been reported only since 1972. In the pages that follow, utilization of hospital, physician, nursing home, and prescription drug services is discussed. In each case rates have been calculated. They will be used later in an attempt to determine changes in the prices of those services.

Two limitations of the data should be noted at the outset. First, they represent bills paid, not services used during the periods in question. If one assumes that the lags between utilization, submission of a claim for payment, and actual payment are relatively constant, or that similar patterns obtain from year to year, then this limitation is unimportant. Second, because a number of states, including some large ones, do not report services used by category of eligibility, the figures presented are incomplete. For each service, however, more than forty states reported in each year. Rates are not likely to have been seriously affected by the omission of several states, but it does mean that it is not possible to compare the number of recipients from year to year from this source because the list of reporting states varies. We will focus, therefore, on the computed rates.

As shown in Table 3–1, the number of users of hospital services increased by 92 percent from 1968 through 1976 and by 23 percent from 1972 through 1976. Further, 15.5 percent of Medicaid recipients used hospital services in 1968, and 14.7 percent used them in 1976, a decline of 0.8 percent. Between 1972 and 1976, the proportion of hospital users among all recipients dropped 1.3 percent (Table 3–2).

Table A–5 shows that there was, overall, a 3.1 percent decline in discharges per 1,000 recipients between 1972 and 1976, from 1,422 to 1,331. Because the nonaged adult categories were combined in 1972, and no data were reported for the small category of blind people, comparisons can be made only from 1973 through 1976. These show that the hospitalization rate for the disabled increased by almost 7 percent, while that for AFDC adults increased by less than one-third of that amount. Rates for the elderly and for children declined by 6.4 percent and 2.2 percent, respectively.

The more revealing figures are those that represent the number of days of care per discharge. The average length of stay declined for each category of eligibles, a reduction of 20.5 percent overall. The reduction for the elderly was more than 22 percent, and for other categories, 7 to 14 percent. The period was marked by some fluctuations within categories, all in a generally downward trend, in contrast to the comparatively greater stability of the discharge rates. Overall, hospital utilization rates declined, both in the rates at which recipients were hospitalized and, particularly, in the length of those hospitalizations.

In physician visits, the period 1972 through 1976 saw a 25 percent increase in the number of recipients who used this service, but a 5 percent drop in the proportion of recipients with visits (Tables 3–1 and 3–2). Overall, there was a 7.3 percent increase in the number of visits per recipient during the period, from 5.5 to 5.7 (Table A–6). This gain was accounted for entirely by the AFDC categories. Visits by children increased from 3.8 in 1972 to 4.4 in 1976, and by AFDC adults, from 6.2 to 6.8. The other adult categories declined: 20.5 percent among the aged, 8.3 percent among the blind, and 5.3 percent among the disabled. Thus, physician utilization in general grew not only in the numbers of people seeing physicians in a year but also in the numbers of visits for the average AFDC-related recipient even though the proportion of Medicaid recipients utilizing physician services declined.

The utilization of skilled nursing facilities and intermediate care facilities exhibited different patterns during the period (Table A–7). While the number of people using SNFs grew by almost 18 percent (Table 3–1), the days of care per recipient dropped by 4.8 percent overall, more for the disabled (8.4 percent) than for the aged (2.7 percent). But the decline was attributable entirely to a drop in 1973, associated with the beginning of ICF coverage. From 1973 through 1976, the rates of use of SNFs increased, but not enough to overcome the large decline in 1973. Data on ICFs are available for the years since 1973 but are reported only for the aged and for all recipients together. The number of recipients using ICFs increased by almost 69 percent in that period, and the number of days per recipient increased by 16 percent (18 percent for the elderly alone). Overall, then, the utilization of extended care facilities has increased by most measures.

In the five years from 1972 through 1976, the numbers of patients obtaining prescribed drugs increased by 30.5 percent. The rate of use increased by a similar amount, from 9.2 prescriptions per recipient to 11.8 (Table A—8). Moreover, the increase in the rate of use was approximately 25 percent for all categories except AFDC adults, which increased by only 14 percent.

Utilization: A Summary

The number of users of services increased for all services between 1972 and 1976. In Chapter 2 we saw that the proportion of eligibles using services also increased. In this chapter we observed that each service had approximately the same proportion of all users at the end of the period as at the beginning; only small changes were discovered in most services. Hospitals, physicians, and drugs were down somewhat. Nursing homes saw the only dramatic increase (87 percent) because of the addition of ICFs as a covered service.

Rates of use were down for most institutional services. Hospital discharges and the number of days per discharge declined from 1972 through 1976, and the number of days of care per recipient in SNFs also declined somewhat. Rates of ICF utilization increased by 16 percent, however; and, when only the period from 1973 through 1976 is considered, days of care per recipient of SNF services increased slightly (2.2 percent), as well.

Rates of use of physician services were up 7 percent overall, but down for the aged, blind, and disabled. Gains of 10 and 16 percent were recorded for AFDC adults and children, respectively. Rates of prescription use also increased.

Thus, for the most part, gains in utilization of services by Medicaid recipients has been accounted for more by spreading benefits over more people than by increasing the utilization of people already in the system. To that extent, therefore, it can be said that one of the goals of the program is being met. But a number of questions relating to utilization remain: What is the quality of the care provided? Are the services appropriate to the patient's physical condition? Are they provided in the most appropriate sites? Is the care comprehensive and continuous or episodic?

In partial response to these questions, several authors have raised doubts about the accessibility and appropriateness of care received by Medicaid recipients. Aday, using a measure that she calls the use-disability index, discovered that, while low-income people with disability averaged more visits to a doctor overall than other income groups, "looking at their use of services relative to their respective need for care . . . it is apparent that the low-income population saw a doctor less often relative to the disability experienced than did the other income groups. This was true both in 1963 and 1970" (Aday, 1976: 223). Davis and Reynolds found similar results for utilization in 1969. They write that "adjustment for health status leads to a striking change in utilization patterns. Instead of following a U-shaped pattern with low-income persons using services more than middle-income persons, utilization increases uniformly with income. Poor persons eligible for welfare use physician services about the same as middle-income persons with comparable health problems, whereas those low-income persons not on public assistance lag substantially behind other poor and middle-income persons in use of services" (Davis and Reynolds, 1976: 397). Kravits and Schneider (1975), using measures of need based on physician assessments of patients' conditions, confirm these findings.

All three sources recognize weaknesses in measures of the need for services. Kravits and Schneider, who used physician ratings of need based on verified diagnoses, come closest to defining these patterns as *under*utilization of services by poor people. Nonetheless, the consistency of the results among the three sources suggests that, although Medicaid has indeed caused poor people to increase their utilization of medical services as intended, income or ability to pay still apparently affects utilization. The extent to which the observed patterns represent a continuing problem depends in part on the stability of the results, on the objectivity of the measures, and on whether utilization by middle- and upper-income individuals is used as the norm.

These questions are not answerable definitely with the evidence currently available. But the utilization data already cited are reassuring enough on the rates of use that the next set of Medicaid utilization questions to be pursued through research should be those relating to the appropriateness, continuity, and quality of the services provided.

THE COST OF CARE REVISITED

In Chapter 2, I attempted to explain the increase in Medicaid expenditures using monthly data because previous studies had shown that the numbers of people eligible for the program had an important influence on utilization and, hence, on costs. It was not possible with those data, however, to resolve the question of the sources of the growth in expenditures. Annual figures on expenditures and utilization rates make it possible to add price to the equation introduced in the previous chapter. Cost and user data were reported for all states, but the rates of utilization that are applied to them were derived from fewer states. In almost all cases, however, at least forty states reported.

Table 3-3.   Annual Expenditures for Medicaid, 1968–1976
(in thousands of dollars)

	1968	1969	1970	1971	1972	1973	1974	1975	1976	Percent Increase 1972-76	Percent Increase 1968-76
A. by Basis of Eligibility											
Aged	1,657,037	1,759,982	1,783,718	2,227,214	1,925,178	3,235,472	3,691,260	4,649,242	5,191,629	169.7	213.3
Blind	30,187	36,120	35,308	47,514	44,511	64,892	79,844	83,466	86,216	93.7	185.6
Disabled	631,957	816,309	994,473	1,235,361	1,353,916	2,015,105	2,388,244	2,873,635	3,549,515	162.2	461.7
AFDC adults	588,309	725,519	892,050	1,116,577	961,919	1,446,083	1,704,418	2,050,210	2,244,947	133.4	281.6
AFDC children	550,236	714,732	841,725	1,092,819	1,139,010	1,426,020	1,694,250	2,013,062	2,352,827	106.6	327.6
Totals	3,742,262	4,325,384	4,805,936	5,939,236	6,299,050	8,639,751	9,982,881	12,292,375	14,134,655	124.4	277.7
B. Type of Service Used											
Gen. hosp.	1,139,485	1,357,379	1,533,676	2,288,384	2,556,687	2,659,507	2,886,921	3,411,389	3,938,303	54.0	245.6
SNF	1,051,538	1,286,175	1,362,092	1,674,000	1,470,939	1,958,938	2,001,861	2,446,173	2,488,376	69.2	136.6
ICF	100,356	—			—	1,059,814	1,584,520	2,215,227	2,790,721	163.3[a]	2,680.8
Physicians	422,179	514,290	616,567	717,104	794,005	925,923	1,083,378	1,247,725	1,388,568	74.9	228.9
Outpt. hosp.	132,505	154,079	221,477	311,048	364,726	267,612	322,010	377,218	556,283	52.5	319.8
Clinic	2,312	12,484	18,200	n.a.	40,939	237,342	284,293	388,825	341,401	733.9	14,666.5
Lab and X-ray	25,631	28,936	31,863	24,769	81,258	104,770	95,942	122,818	177,055	117.9	590.8
Prescr. drugs	280,918	347,973	403,194	473,020	511,877	609,338	712,562	832,173	957,035	87.0	240.7
All	3,742,262	4,325,384	4,808,360	5,939,236	6,299,050	8,639,751	9,982,881	12,292,375	14,134,655	124.4	277.7

Source: National Center for Social Statistics (later, Health Care Financing Administration), Report B-4 for 1968–1976, except Report B-5 for 1971. Totals include estimates for nonreporting states.
[a]Calculated for the period 1973–1976.

Table 3–4. Expenditures by Category as a Proportion of all Expenditures

(in percent)

	1968	1969	1970	1971	1972	1973	1974	1975	1976	Percent Change 1972–1976	Percent Change 1968–1976
A. By Basis of Eligibility											
Aged	44.3	40.7	37.1	37.5	30.6	37.4	37.0	37.8	36.7	6.1	−7.6
Blind	0.8	0.8	0.7	0.8	0.7	0.8	0.8	0.7	0.6	−0.1	−0.2
Disabled	16.9	18.8	20.7	20.8	21.5	23.3	23.9	23.4	25.1	3.6	8.2
AFDC adults	15.7	16.8	18.6	18.8	15.3	16.7	17.1	16.7	15.9	0.6	0.2
AFDC children	14.7	16.5	17.5	18.4	18.1	16.5	17.0	16.4	16.6	−1.5	1.9
Total	92.4	93.6	94.6	96.3	86.2	94.7	95.8	95.0	94.9	2.5	8.7
B. By Type of Service Used											
Gen. hosp.	30.4	31.4	31.9	38.5	40.6	30.8	28.9	27.8	27.9	−12.7	−2.5
SNF	28.1	29.7	28.3	28.2	23.4	22.7	20.1	19.9	17.6	−5.8	−10.5
ICF	2.7	—	—	—	—	12.3	15.9	18.0	19.7	19.7	17.0
Physicians	11.3	11.9	12.8	12.1	12.6	10.7	10.9	10.2	9.8	−2.8	−1.5
Outpt. hosp.	3.5	3.6	4.6	5.2	5.8	3.1	3.2	3.1	3.9	−1.9	0.4
Clinic	10.06	0.3	0.4	n.a.	0.6	2.7	2.8	3.2	2.4	1.8	2.4
Lab and X-ray	0.7	0.7	0.7	0.4	1.3	1.2	0.9	0.9	1.3	—	0.6
Prescr. drugs	7.5	8.0	8.4	8.0	8.1	7.1	7.1	6.8	6.8	−1.3	−0.7

Source: National Center for Social Statistics (later, Health Care Financing Administration), Report B-4 for 1968–1976, except Report B-5 for 1971. Totals include estimates for nonreporting states.

Annual Medicaid Expenditures

Tables 3–3 and 3–4 reveal that expenditures grew by 277.7 percent between 1968 and 1976 and by 124.4 percent between 1972 and 1976. They grew least for the blind and aged among the eligibility categories and for SNFs, hospitals, physicians, outpatient hospital services, and prescription drugs among the services. Most of the large proportional increase was accounted for by the prodigious growth in expenditures for ICF services. In almost all cases, the increase in expenditures was three to four times as great as the growth in number of users. Finally, the only categories to increase their share of expenditures were the aged and disabled among the eligibility categories and ICFs among the services. All were related in that the elderly and disabled are the principal users of ICF services.

Average expenditures per recipient were calculated on the basis of eligibility and type of service used (see Table 3–5). For all recipients, average expenditures increased by 66.6 percent from 1972 through 1976. While there is considerable variation in rates among the categories, the proportional increase in expenditures per recipient was much less than the proportional increase in expenditures by themselves and also less than the percentage increase in number of users of services. Average expenditures for the aged and the blind increased more than the overall average, and those for AFDC adults and children increased less.

One conclusion to be drawn is that ICFs had a disproportionate effect on all aspects of the program: utilization, expenditures, and expenditures per recipient.

Prices for Selected Services

Returning to the equation presented in Chapter 2, which shows the relation of expenditures, rates of utilization, and price, we can now calculate the average price of several of the major services provided under Medicaid.[c] Table 3–6 shows that prices for all services increased during the period 1972 through 1976 and that some increased more than others. The cost of a day in the hospital increased considerably more than others. The price of a physician visit increased proportionally only half as much as a day in the hospital. The price of a day in an ICF increased by 36 percent (though this was over four years, whereas the other changes were calculated over a five-year period). The average price of a prescription increased least of all, only 9.5 percent over the five years.

---

[c]Although for convenience I refer to price, expenditure per unit of service is a more precise term.

Table 3-5.   Average Expenditures per Recipient 1968-1976
(in dollars)

	1968	1969	1970	1971	1972	1973	1974	1975	1976	Percent Increase 1972-1976	1968-1976
A. By Basis of Eligibility											
Aged	603.22	613.23	505.45	618.67	563.41	911.66	970.11	1,256.89	1,363.35	142.0	126.0
Blind	471.67	368.57	320.98	386.29	408.36	636.20	587.09	780.06	879.76	115.4	86.5
Disabled	750.54	790.23	694.46	823.57	809.27	1,093.38	1,047.48	1,245.08	1,332.40	64.6	77.5
AFDC adults	264.05	231.65	262.99	237.57	300.98	348.79	377.84	439.77	428.59	42.4	62.3
AFDC children	98.71	109.67	116.23	131.66	139.29	161.57	174.13	205.92	221.03	58.7	123.9
Totals	306.89	296.02	292.71	307.37	343.98	432.01	453.58	548.45	573.04	66.6	86.7
B. By Type of Service Used											
Gen. hosp.	604.82	610.88	603.33		871.10	803.96	859.46	978.88	1,089.74	25.1	80.2
SNF	1,943.61	2,225.22	2,304.72		2,617.33	2,843.16	2,961.33	3,926.44	3,912.54	49.5	101.3
ICF	1,497.85	—	—		—	2,254.92	2,460.43	3,111.27	3,523.64	56.3[a]	135.2
Physicians	55.58	56.66	59.19		62.53	68.68	70.87	80.75	87.21	39.5	56.9
Outpt. hosp.	50.46	46.96	53.61		66.47	50.53	56.50	62.13	74.69	12.4	48.0
Clinic	22.89	23.03	30.59		78.58	119.81	132.41	159.94	151.40	92.7	561.4
Lab and X-ray	28.17	21.20	21.00		22.40	25.77	23.00	27.96	35.45	58.3	25.8
Prescr. drugs	41.19	40.77	40.90		44.43	49.63	49.00	59.15	63.63	43.2	54.5
All	306.89	296.02	292.85		343.98	432.01	453.58	548.45	573.04	66.6	86.7

Source: Tables 3-1 and 3-2.
[a]Calculated for the period 1973-1976.

Table 3–6. Average Price per Unit of Service, Selected Eligibility Categories, 1972–1976[a]

	1972	1973	1974	1975	1976	Percent Change 1972–1976
Per Hospital Day						
Aged	18.75	15.53[b]	11.48[c]	16.51	24.86	32.6
Disabled	—	101.32	94.75	103.41	108.45	7.0[d]
AFDC adults	—	93.96	100.36	117.14	141.37	50.5[d]
AFDC children	74.90	90.64	92.47	111.56	134.82	80.0
All	60.18	77.98	79.21	80.23	98.45	63.6
Per Physician Visit						
Aged	6.08	6.71	7.67	9.20	10.17	67.3
Blind	11.27	11.73	13.04	14.03	15.64	38.8
Disabled	13.27	14.64	15.50	17.29	17.89	34.8
AFDC adults	14.63	16.57	16.61	16.84	17.94	22.6
AFDC children	11.43	10.99	12.50	16.78	14.07	23.1
All	11.34	12.36	13.25	14.72	15.04	32.6
Per Day in SNF						
Aged	13.47	12.52	12.80	16.04	15.67	16.3
Disabled	13.82	14.39	13.98	19.74	19.55	41.5
All	13.49	12.88	13.07	16.70	16.44	21.9
Per Day in ICF						
Aged	—	9.41	9.60	11.38	12.29	30.6[d]
All	—	9.28	9.54	11.66	12.62	36.0[d]
Per Prescription						
Aged	4.80	4.78	4.92	5.19	5.69	18.5
Blind	5.29	5.18	3.71	5.51	5.94	12.3
Disabled	5.27	5.09	5.41	5.57	6.08	15.4
AFDC adults	4.74	4.58	4.61	4.83	5.32	12.2
AFDC children	3.93	3.48	3.81	4.30	4.10	4.3
All	4.95	4.78	5.47	5.45	5.42	9.5

[a] Calculated from NCSS (later, HCFA) Report B-4 and B-4 Supplements, 1972–1976. These data reflect reports from more than forty states in each instance except for the two noted.
[b] 1973 aged calculated on the basis of data from nineteen states.
[c] 1974 aged calculated on the basis of data from twenty-nine states.
[d] Calculated for 1973–1976.

It should be noted that the payment for a hospital day for the elderly appears to be very low, especially when compared with a hospital day for other groups. Undoubtedly, the difference is explained by the fact that much of the hospital cost incurred by the elderly is paid for by Medicare. To a considerable extent, therefore, the Medicaid share covers the deductible and coinsurance since the average length of stay is well below the limit covered by Medicare.

Except for hospital days, where the increase in the payment per day was 9.6 percent higher than the increase in expenditures, the increase in prices for 1972 through 1976 for the major services was substantially less than increases in expenditures. For hospitals, the rates of utilization declined so substantially that the amount of the increase attributable to price was larger than for other services, in which utilization did not decline or declined less sharply (see Table 3—7).

Thus, since the average number of physician visits per person increased somewhat, the contribution of price to the growth in expenditures for physician services was less than that for hospital services. And since the number of prescriptions filled for the average recipient increased so markedly, the amount of the increase attributable to price was still less than that for physicians.

The question remains why expenditures for some services increased more because of price changes while those for others grew because of increased utilization rates and still others because of larger numbers of users. To answer this question, we must ask some others: How were the various providers paid and how did this change during the period from 1972 through 1976? Were prices more likely to be limited in some cases than in others? If so, did the providers affected by these limits respond by increasing the quantity of services provided to the average recipient more than providers not faced with price limitations? The Canadian experience, for example, shows that when physician fees were fixed, patients received more physician services, and physician income did not decline (see Marmor, 1975).

In the case of Medicaid, other factors beyond the scope of the program may also have an effect. For example, during the early seventies there was much greater use of generic prescriptions than previously, which may account in part for the relatively small price increases in prescription drugs. If that indeed is part of the explanation, did pharmacists compensate by dividing prescriptions in order to collect additional fees? If they did, that practice would have contributed to lowering the average prescription price, too, since the amount of the drug provided in each prescription would have been

Table 3–7.   Percent Change in Recipients, Expenditures, and Price, Selected Years

	Recipients		Expenditures		Average Expenditures per Recipient		Average Price per Unit of Service
	1972–1976	1968–1976	1972–1976	1968–1976	1972–1976	1968–1976	1972–1976
Aged	11.4	38.6	169.7	213.3	142.0	126.0	
Blind	−10.1	53.1	93.7	185.6	115.4	86.5	
Disabled	59.2	216.4	162.2	461.7	64.6	77.5	
AFDC adults	32.6	135.1	133.4	281.6	42.4	62.3	
AFDC children	30.2	91.0	106.6	327.6	58.7	123.9	
All	34.7	102.3	124.4	277.7	66.6	86.7	
Gen. hosp.	23.1	91.8	54.0	245.6	25.1	80.2	63.6
SNF	13.2	17.6	69.2	136.6	49.5	101.3	21.9
ICF	68.5[a]	—	163.3[a]	—	56.3[a]	—	36.0[a]
Physicians	25.4	109.6	74.9	228.9	39.5	56.9	32.6
Outpt. hosp.	35.7	183.6	52.5	319.8	12.4	48.0	
Clinic	332.8	2,132.7	733.9	14,666.5	92.7	561.4	
Lab and X-ray	37.7	4,489.0	117.9	590.8	58.3	25.8	
Prescr. drugs	30.5	120.5	87.0	240.7	43.2	54.5	9.5
All	34.7	102.3	124.4	277.7	66.6	86.7	

[a]1973–1976.

smaller than if the physician's entire order had been filled at once. The large increase in the rate of utilization supports both hypotheses.

A caveat should be entered. These calculations assume that the content of the services remained constant throughout the period. Undoubtedly, that was not entirely true. The particular services provided by hospitals, for example, depend to a considerable extent on the mix of diagnoses among hospitalized patients. Since that mix changes from year to year, it can be expected to alter the nature of hospital services provided. Changes in medical technology also affect prices and outlays, probably by tending to increase both. Medicine is one industry in which improvements in techniques usually result in cost increases, rather than savings through greater efficiency (see Feldstein, 1971) because of the required new capital equipment or the specially trained personnel.

CONCLUSION

The amount to be spent on Medicaid services is a political matter. It is determined in part by the answers to such questions as how keen is competition with other programs for public funds? And can the additional revenues needed be raised without raising tax rates? If policymakers want to try to limit expenditures, they will be more likely to succeed if their decisions reflect an understanding of how decisions to utilize services are made. For example, since, as we saw earlier in this chapter, patients exercise their greatest control over utilization when they decide whether to enter the medical care system, policies which depend on patients for their effect should focus on the decision to seek care in the first place; and those that depend on physicians should aim for an impact on the amount and sites of services for patients who have already sought their help.

In deciding which set of decisions to try to alter, policymakers need to examine what data reveal about the sources of Medicaid expenditure increases. We saw in this chapter that the growth in outlays appears to be accounted for more by increases in the volume of services used by recipients than by rising prices, for example. Moreover, the increased utilization is attributable partly to growth in the number of users of services and partly to the quantity of services used by each.

In the next several chapters, aspects of the Medicaid program that affect utilization decisions will be taken up. First, I present material on the eligibility criteria that determine who may use services paid for by Medicaid; then, in Chapter 5, I take up the benefit structure, which determines which services and how many of each providers may offer to patients under the program. In Chapter 6, I focus on the methods of compensating providers. And, in Chapter 7, state efforts at the monitoring and direct control of utilization are discussed. All of these factors can, theoretically at least, influence patterns of utilization and provision of services that have implications not only for the health of patients, but also for expenditures under the Medicaid program. In each case, the focus is on those Medicaid decisions made by state policymakers that, by setting the conditions of the program, influence decisions by the two other principal parties to Medicaid, the patient and the provider.

One final word about the enterprise. While it is reasonable to encourage scrutiny of utilization decisions by those who make them (providers as well as patients and their families) and also by those who pay for them, investigators should not embark on such an undertaking with the assumption that they will find widespread overuse—whether deliberately for personal gain or inadvertent. Nor should they assume that large financial savings would result even if some care decisions can be altered without harm to individuals. Medicaid has become a multibillion dollar program, and it is naive to expect that programmatic adjustments will result in substantial dollar savings nationally. The reasons are that Medicaid is really fifty programs, not just one, and that actors in the Medicaid and medical care systems are likely to adapt in ways that would maintain the balance among the parts. Yet if policy decisions can be identified that would control the rate of increase in expenditures without denying poor people the care they need, something of value will have been accomplished.

Eligibility

Chapter 3 established that the number of people eligible for Medicaid benefits has grown substantially since the program's inception. That point is placed in the context of growth of the total U.S. population in Table 4–1. The table shows, for example, that, although the number of children under the age of eighteen declined by almost 8 percent between 1968 and 1976, the number of individuals eligible for Medicaid benefits under the Aid to Families with Dependent Children (AFDC) category grew by almost 84 percent in the same period. Almost all of that growth had occurred by 1972, and the number of AFDC eligibles remained remarkably constant after 1972. In contrast, while the elderly population grew by 20 percent, the number of elderly public assistance recipients increased by only 6 percent, most of which coincided with the changeover from the state-administered Old Age Assistance program to the federally run Supplemental Security Income (SSI) program. Overall, the numbers of Medicaid eligibles, including the medically needy, grew as a proportion of the American population by a little more than 3 percent between 1968 and 1976.

Eligibility for benefits affects expenditures differently for the categorically eligible and the medically needy. Assuming relatively constant rates of illness among categorical eligibles, utilization of each service (and, hence, expenditures) will increase as the number of eligibles increases because those illness rates will apply to more people. Thus, when we consider the categorically eligible, we focus first on the numbers of eligibles by state and then on their rates of utilization. The medically needy, in contrast, become eligible for services at the point of utilization. That is, their eligibility is determined when

Table 4-1.　U.S. Population by Age and Medicaid Eligibles by Category, 1966–1976

	U.S. Population (000)				Medicaid Eligibles (000)						Medicaid Eligibles as Percent of Population
	Total	Under 18[a]	18–64	65+	Total	OAA	Blind	Disabled	AFDC	Medically Needy	
1976	214,659	65,190	126,535	22,934	21,662	2,148	76	2,012	11,181	6,245	10.1
1974	211,390	67,262	122,312	21,815	20,398	2,286	75	1,636	11,006	5,395	9.6
1972	209,042	68,628	119,275	21,139	19,275	1,933	80	1,169	11,069	5,024	9.2
1970	203,165	69,653	113,462	20,050	16,983	2,082	81	935	9,659	4,226	8.4
1968	199,861	70,809	109,923	19,129	13,782	2,027	81	702	6,086	4,886[b]	6.9
1966	195,857	70,665	106,736	18,457	—	2,073	81	588	4,666	—	—
					Percent Change						
1974–76	1.5	-3.1	3.5	5.1	6.2	-6.0	1.3	23.0	1.6	15.8	
1972–74	1.1	-2.0	2.5	3.2	5.8	18.3	-6.3	39.9	-0.6	7.4	
1970–72	2.9	-1.5	5.1	5.4	13.5	-7.2	-1.2	25.0	14.6	18.9	
1968–70	1.7	-1.6	3.2	4.8	23.2	2.7	n.c.	33.2	58.7	—	
1966–68	2.0	0.2	3.0	3.6	—	—	—	—	—	—	
1968–1976	7.4	-7.9	15.1	19.9	57.2	6.0	-6.2	186.6	83.7	—	

Sources: Public Aid Recipients (OAA, Blind, Disabled, AFDC): 1966, 1968, 1970, *Historical Statistics of the U.S., Part I*, page 356; 1972, 1974, 1976, *Statistical Abstract of the U.S.*, 1977, table 543, p. 345 (as of December of each year). Both published by U.S. Government Printing Office. Medically Needy Recipients: *Medicaid: Recipients, Payments, and Services*, Annual Reports B-4, table 1. Published by USDHEW, Health Care Financing Administration. U.S. Population: *Statistical Abstract of the U.S.*, 1967, 1969, 1971, 1973, 1974, 1975, 1977. Table: Population by Age, States, Figures for 1972 were estimated by attributing half of the difference between 1971 and 1973 to 1972.

[a] Age groupings are meant to be roughly comparable to public assistance categories. OAA is comparable to 65 and over; 18—64 is comparable to the adult categories; and under 18 is comparable to AFDC. It should be noted, however-er, that people are eligible for AFDC benefits in some states until age 21 and that the AFDC column includes adults who are eligible under that category.

[b] Medically Needy totals for 1968 do not include data for Colorado or Pennsylvania.

(or after) they seek services. Thus their overall utilization rate is 100 percent, although for specific services it will obviously be less then 100 percent. Therefore, when we consider the eligibility factor as it relates to the medically needy, we focus on changes in the numbers of medically needy users of services by state and the number and types of services used.

Thus the categorically eligible may use services when the need arises, but some will have no need for medical care; and *all* of the medically needy will use services during the period of their eligibility. Because the decisions affecting eligibility (as well as covered services, payment of providers, and other factors) vary from state to state, the analysis for this and several succeeding chapters is shifted to the state level. The categorically eligible and the medically needy are treated separately. But before turning to that analysis, I describe the process by which a person or family becomes eligible for Medicaid benefits. Although procedures vary in their details, the fundamental process is the same from state to state.

THE PROCESS

A person becomes eligible for Medicaid benefits by qualifying under one of several categories: Aid to Families with Dependent Children, Supplemental Security Income or, in those states that cover them, Medically Needy.

Aid to Families with Dependent Children is a federally assisted, state-administered public assistance program under which eligibility determination and maintenance is a state responsibility carried out under federal regulations. These regulations require, among other things, that applications be taken promptly; that they be written (although in the event of incapacitation, the applicants themselves need not complete the forms); that applicants be fully informed about their rights and obligations and that specific written materials be available for the purpose; that reasons for decisions be specified; and that redeterminations be done at least annually and more often if information indicating a change in eligibility status comes to the agency. Beyond these minimum standards, there is considerable room for state variability. Moreover, it is not clear to what extent the minimum standards are met by the states' actual procedures. And finally, the specific income and resource criteria, as well as optional factors, are left to the states to decide.

The Supplemental Security Income eligibility process, by contrast, is a responsibility of the Social Security Administration (SSA), although in some states it is performed by the state under contract to SSA. Medicaid eligibility remains a state responsibility, however, in all cases. Since Medicaid eligibility is no longer auto-matic—at the state's option—under SSI[a] separate Medicaid eligibility determinations must be made in those states in which Medicaid eligibility prior to SSI was pegged at a level below that of current SSI payments. At their option, then, the states may choose not to cover such people or to cover them as medically needy or under spend-down provisions. In each such case, data not obtained in the SSI eligibility process may be required. Moreover, the SSA data tape itself is important, and problems have arisen with its reliability, accuracy, and timeliness.

Title XIX also permits states at their option to use federal funds for part of the cost of medical assistance for certain people who do not receive public assistance grants. The medically needy as defined in the law would qualify for one of the federal public assistance categories except for the fact that their income exceeds the state's income eligibility limits by less than 133.33 percent of the maximum amount paid by the state for AFDC families of comparable size. If states choose to exercise this option, they must follow the procedural rules specified by federal regulations for AFDC eligibility.

Two additional points about Medicaid eligibility are important to this discussion. First, income is not the only criterion. Recipients of cash assistance and Medicaid benefits must also meet any family composition, employment status, and assets test applicable in a state under AFDC or SSI rules. To illustrate: federal regulations governing SSI eligibility permit individuals to retain $1,500 in personal property and a home with a market value of up to $25,000. Some states have established more restrictive criteria on personal property, automobiles, and houses, as well as limitations on the transfer of property.

Second, the process of "spending down" must also be understood. In most instances, individuals establish eligibility for benefits under the medically needy provisions when they have need for medical services. To do that they must, as noted, demonstrate that their assets fall within the prescribed limits. They must also show either that their incomes are below the maximum or that they have incurred sufficient medical expenses to reduce their incomes to the eligibility level. The latter method of demonstrating income eligibility, called "spending down," is a complex process that varies from state to state in several important ways. For example, in defining "incurred" medical expenses, some states require that money actually be spent, while others insist only that a debt be established. Moreover, although federal regulations permit states to consider as income funds

---

[a] See the section on the medically needy later in this chapter.

expected to be received during the next six months, some states have established shorter periods.[b]

Finally, all states using a more restricted standard for Medicaid eligibility—even those that have no program for the medically needy—must permit SSI recipients to establish their eligibility for Medicaid benefits by spending down. We will return to this factor in our discussion of the medically needy elderly later in this chapter.

The eligibility determination process is activated by an application for benefits. The application may be initiated by clients when they apply for AFDC, by the SSI program when it notifies the state's Medicaid staff that a state resident is eligible for SSI, by a hospital or other provider, by a patient who appears for services without being able to demonstrate the ability to pay for them, or as the result of the program's outreach efforts.

The "appearance" to apply for assistance need not be in person. Some states, particularly when no income maintenance grant is involved, make it possible for potential clients to complete necessary forms over the telephone or in places other than a public assistance office (e.g., a hospital in which the applicant is a patient). This situation is another example of the need to recognize that Medicaid is both a health and a welfare program.

Patients may have social workers in the hospital in which they are receiving care initiate the application for them. The completed forms in this way are then submitted to the program and proceed through the steps leading to a decision regarding eligibility. These procedures make the application process less burdensome for the patient, encourage more applications, and increase the likelihood that the provider—which, in such situations is most often a hospital or nursing facility—will be paid for the services provided.

Any process requires time. The amount of time required in an eligibility determination process depends heavily on the amount of information required of the applicant, the ease with which it can be produced, and the nature of the review performed upon it. The first two items, in turn, are largely a function of the state's criteria for eligibility. These criteria generally fall into three categories:

1. Categorical relatedness
2. Income
3. Other resources.

These are discussed in turn, as is a fourth important determinant of the time involved in the eligibility process—forms and procedures.

[b] For a more complete discussion of spending down, see Davidson et al. (1980: Chapter 4).

Categorical relatedness

It is to the state's advantage to include its potential Medicaid recipients under one of the federally assisted categories in order to receive federal matching funds for the benefits themselves (administrative costs are shared by the federal government even for other categories of eligibles). Women applying for assistance under the AFDC category (and men in those states which cover them) must establish that they have children and that the children fall into the eligible age range, which varies from state to state. The nature of the mother's relationship to the children's father must be established; only twenty-seven states and the District of Columbia will cover a family with an unemployed father present. It must be established too, that the children are dependent, which, like other factors, is defined by each state. In some, dependency is assumed by virtue of the children's being very young and living apart from their father. In others, dependency is related to deprivation, which may be defined, for example, in terms of the mother's absence from the home for a specified period (e.g., spending thirty days in a hospital). Finally, states have rules regarding the responsibility of various relatives for the care of the children. In some, parents, if they can be found and are employable, are responsible for the care of their children who are under twenty-one. They may be responsible, as well, for adult children who are applying under SSI provisions because of blindness or permanent disability. These requirements mean that before individuals can establish eligibility for public assistance—and, hence, for Medicaid—benefits, they must establish either that they have no responsible relatives or that their relatives are too poor (again, defined by the state) to assume that responsibility with their own resources.

All of these criteria demand information. An applicant must be able to answer the questions on the application form, usually asked by an eligibility worker in a local public assistance office, and provide data in condiderable detail. Moreover, he or she must be able to verify some or all of the major data elements. For example, if age is a requirement of the category, a birth certificate or derivative document must be presented. The lack of such documentation will delay the establishment of eligibility and may even defeat it. Such requirements affect the efficiency and the accuracy of the process since the documentation may not be readily available to the applicant and since, whenever it is presented, the information must be evaluated.

Income

Public assistance is a means-tested program. Eligibility can be established only if applicants who meet other criteria can demonstrate

Table 4-2.   Annual Need and Payment Standard for an AFDC Family of Two and an AFDC Family of Four, as of October 1, 1978

State	2-Person Family		4-Person Family		State	2-Person Family		4-Person Family	
	Need	Payment	Need	Payment		Need	Payment	Need	Payment
Alabama	$1,728	$1,200	$2,880	$2,040	Montana	1,956	1,956	3,024	3,024
Alaska	3,600	3,600	4,800	4,800	Nebraska	2,760	2,520	3,960	3,528
Arizona	2,160	1,512	3,384	2,364	Nevada	2,748	2,004	4,104	3,000
Arkansas	2,448	1,596	3,492	2,268					
California	3,384	3,096	5,064	4,548	New Hampshire	1,656	1,656	2,652	2,652
					New Jersey	2,820	2,820	4,272	4,272
Colorado	2,160	2,160	3,312	3,312	New Mexico	1,920	1,656	2,868	2,472
Connecticut	2,904	2,904	4,188	4,188	New York	3,708	3,708	5,376	5,376
Delaware	2,172	2,172	3,444	3,444	North Carolina	1,908	1,908	2,400	2,400
District of Columbia	2,712	2,436	4,188	3,768					
Florida	1,800	1,428	2,760	2,184	North Dakota	2,640	2,640	4,164	4,164
					Ohio	3,408	2,016	5,172	3,048
Georgia	1,932	936	2,724	1,776	Oklahoma	2,196	2,196	3,408	3,408
Guam	2,412	2,412	3,672	3,672	Oregon	3,516	3,204	4,752	4,320
Hawaii	4,440	4,440	6,168	6,168	Pennsylvania	3,120	3,120	4,476	4,476
Idaho	3,528	3,072	4,740	4,128					
Illinois	2,448	2,448	3,600	3,600	Puerto Rico	948	384	1,512	600
					Rhode Island	3,060	3,060	4,308	4,308
Indiana	2,964	1,800	4,356	3,000	South Carolina	1,656	900	2,604	1,404
Iowa	2,808	2,664	4,512	4,284	South Dakota	3,024	3,024	3,996	3,996
Kansas	2,592	2,592	3,060	3,060	Tennessee	1,704	1,188	2,604	1,572
Kentucky	1,620	1,620	2,820	2,820					
Louisiana	1,416	1,104	2,436	1,896	Texas	1,380	1,032	2,244	1,680
					Utah	3,372	2,592	5,196	3,996
Maine	2,460	2,088	4,188	3,564	Vermont	4,260	3,108	3,988	4,368
Maryland	2,436	1,872	3,768	2,904	Virgin Islands	1,104	1,104	1,992	1,992
Massachusetts	2,928	2,928	4,164	4,164	Virginia	2,088	1,884	3,264	2,940
Michigan	3,468	3,468	5,016	5,016					
Minnesota	3,264	3,264	4,620	4,620	Washington	3,240	3,240	4,620	4,620
					West Virginia	2,628	1,968	3,984	2,988
Mississippi	2,460	360	3,324	720	Wisconsin	3,960	3,600	5,592	5,088
Missouri	3,000	1,200	4,380	2,040	Wyoming	2,520	2,520	3,240	3,240

Source: Institute for Medicaid Management, *Data on the Medicaid Program: Eligibility, Services, Expenditures, Fiscal Years 1966–78* (USDHEW/HCFA/Medicaid Bureau, 1978), pp. 79–80.

Note: All amounts are rounded to next highest dollar amount.

that they are poor enough to qualify. The central questions regarding income eligibility are: At what level of income should eligibility be established? (How poor does a family need to be?) What constitutes income? And what evidence shall be necessary to demonstrate that level of income?

Table 4–2 shows the variation in eligible-income level by state. Three states set the annual need standards for a family of four under the AFDC program at less than $2,500, and nine set it at more than $4,800. Some of the discrepancy can be attributed to differences in cost of living, but much remains to be explained in other ways.[c]

Once the income limits are established, the question becomes, what is income? To answer this question we must ask several others. What is the unit being evaluated: individual, family, household? Should the state consider gross income or net income? If the latter, what types of income need to be counted and what kinds can be disgarded? For example, how much and what types of work-related expenditures should be counted in computing net income?[d]

Finally the question becomes, how much and what kinds of evidence are sufficient to make the eligibility determination? A statement from an employer or a payroll check stub might be acceptable for employed applicants. But some of these may be paid in cash, and others will be unemployed. How can the incomes of such persons, perhaps subsisting on irregular payments from former husbands or from relatives, be verified? That it is difficult to do so is obvious. What are the states' incentives for pushing hard? If, on the one hand, they are able to establish an applicant's eligibility for a federally assisted category, the federal government will share the costs. If, on the other hand, they are unable to establish an applicant's eligibility for such a category, they may be forced to absorb 100 percent of the cost when the applicant applies for state- or locally funded general assistance. In other words, the easier the states' procedures, the more likely they are to receive federal help, which means that the states have an incentive to establish an applicant's eligibility. Thus, if an applicant claims an income that would make him or her eligible but cannot verify it, the state may not push too hard in order to avoid being saddled with the entire assistance and medical care cost burden. Of course, there is the chance that the applicant denied benefits may not apply for general assistance and may not need medical serv-

---

[c] These, however, are beyond the scope of this book.

[d] This question raises equity issues. For instance, if transportation costs are disregarded for the worker who qualifies for assistance by virtue of a larger family, is it fair that a better-paid co-worker must count them as income? But if they are not disregarded, the incentive to work, and thus to escape the welfare rolls, is reduced.

ices. In either of the latter events, the state would save still more by denying any benefits.

Other resources

The comments regarding income apply equally to criteria concerning other resources. Variations among the states can be illustrated by reference to California and Washington, which, though close in geography, are far apart in their treatment of applicants' resources. In 1970, applicants under the medically needy programs in both states were permitted to retain homes they already owned as well as household furnishings. Other personal property was limited to $1,500 for an individual and up to $3,000 for a family of two or more in California; but in Washington the limits were $750 for an individual, $1,450 for a family of two, and another $50 for each additional family member. In some states, like New York, the transfer of real property within a specified period (which varies with the state) is assumed to be for the purposes of establishing eligibility for public assistance and, therefore, is not allowed.

Forms and procedures

As noted earlier, applicants usually appear at local public assistance offices to apply for cash grants and/or Medicaid benefits. There they come into contact with eligibility workers, who usually are at least high-school graduates. In many cases the workers are only a step or two removed from assistance themselves, and that fact may color their attitudes toward clients. The workers are important actors in the entire process, for they must not only obtain information necessary to the eligibility decision, which, as indicated, is not always easy, but they must also exercise considerable judgment about both the adequacy of that information and the eligibility verdict itself.

Training of workers is critical. They perform under considerable pressure from a variety of sources. One is the waiting line of applicants. Federal regulations require that applicants receive prompt attention, but the fact is that they often must wait days if not weeks for initial appointments. Other pressures include complaints from the federal government and/or the media that some applicants are erroneously declared eligible and the demands of superiors to toughen the process in order to reduce the number of approvals and, thereby, the amount of welfare benefits distributed. The result often works hardships on applicants. An example is the seventeen-year-old girl, three months pregnant, who had to return four times to a public aid office in her home city before she could even see a worker. When he finally did hear her request, the worker told her, without justification, that she was ineligible for benefits. It took several additional weeks and the intervention of a persistent social worker from a voluntary social agency for this girl's formal application to be taken. In the meantime, the girl had become depressed and appeared to her social worker to be on the verge of a breakdown. She had recently lost her widowed mother, was pregnant with her first child, and was bleeding so that the pregnancy was threatened (Davidson, 1974). Many applicants are discouraged from returning by workers who say prematurely and with no good basis in fact that the applicants are not likely to be judged eligible anyway and so should not apply.

Public assistance workers engage in a number of practices like those in the illustration, which raise public policy issues: how to achieve effective administrative control of the eligibility determination process; how to provide equitable (not to mention sympathetic) treatment of people in need; and how to comply with federal regulations which, in some instances, prohibit these practices. It would seem to make sense, for example, that workers be required to accept all applications, make appointments at the earliest possible time to take those applications, and make the determination of eligibility on the basis of information in the applications themselves. Further, when an application is denied, the regulation under which the denial is made should be cited by the worker. These two reasonable suggestions are probably required by federal regulations, which say:

> Applicants will be informed about the eligibility requirements and their rights and obligations under the program. Under this requirement individuals are given information in written form, and orally, as appropriate, about coverage, conditions of eligibility, scope of the program, and related services available. (45CFR206.10)

Yet federal officials are unable to monitor local performance systematically.

The presence of federal and state regulations and their form is another source of pressure on eligibility workers. The regulations supposedly provide decision rules to guide the collection of information and the determinations based on it. In some cases, however, the rules are vague and require considerable worker discretion in interpreting them. In other cases, they attempt to be so specific as to cover every possible situation. Not only can they rarely, if ever, do that, but also they become so detailed that it is difficult to find the precisely applicable rule even if it exists. The result, in addition to adding time to the process, is greater inequity, resulting from the varying care and patience with which workers search the regulations.

Another pressure on workers is the length and difficulty of the forms they must complete. In New York State, the application form is eleven pages long and requires an interview approaching two hours to finish (see copy in appendix).

Training is important not only because the eligibility workers operate under pressure but also because to complete the application forms conscientiously is a difficult task at best. Workers need to learn how to follow up on information provided and how to recognize and check on inconsistencies (as when, for example, the applicant claims no income but pays $200 rent each month). The largest cause of erroneous eligibility decisions is misinformation provided by the applicant, much of it unintentional. The evaluation can be based only on what the client says, and if the worker does not obtain sufficient information on which to base an accurate decision, the chance of error increases. But training is often perfunctory, turnover high, and supervision erratic; the results undoubtedly reflect these conditions.

Once the information is received from the applicant, it must be assessed so that an eligibility determination can be made. To what extent do state personnel perform independent verifications of the data provided by applicants, whose principal interest, after all, is to establish their eligibility? Do they verify all data provided by all applicants? Do they check only some? Do they sample applicants randomly? Clearly the answers to these questions have direct implications for the efficiency and effectiveness of the system in making accurate, timely decisions. To check all applications takes time and money; to sample applications takes less of both. Are the decisions produced by the two approaches qualitatively different? What is the impact on the cost of the benefits provided? Are more people who are truly ineligible approved under one method of verification than another? How many such people are approved erroneously, and how much money does it cost? Similarly, how many are inappropriately denied benefits because, although the information obtained was inaccurate, the errors escaped detection by inadequate verification procedures?

Two other important aspects of the eligibility determination and management system are the speed with which the determinations, once made, are transmitted to clients and to providers, and the accessibility of relevant staff to accurate, complete lists of eligibles. The use of computers may help in these areas, but two questions arise: To what extent do states use them at all as part of the eligibility process? And to what extent is their full potential realized?

The Medicaid Management Information System (MMIS) and other computer-based management tools require eligibility data so that providers can determine, in some cases at the point of service, whether a patient is eligible for benefits; and, later on, so that the claims payment staff can determine that a patient was in fact eligible on the day he or she received services. States vary in their use of computers, however, and have been slow to adopt the comprehensive, but complicated, MMIS.

Before leaving the subject of eligibility determination, we must take note of the fact that federal regulations specify that eligibility files be updated periodically. AFDC cases must be reexamined every six months, and other categories, including medical assistance, annually. To what extent are these requirements actually met? When redeterminations are made, what is the effect on the rolls? Is the net number of eligibles reduced, and, if so, by how much? Do former eligibles return to the rolls later on, and, if so, to what degree? Are some categories more stable than others? The federal regulations imply that AFDC eligibility is less stable than the other categories, but is that conclusion warranted? A substantial proportion of SSI recipients are elderly and, thus, have a higher mortality rate than the younger eligibles in other categories. When redeterminations are done, how do the procedures followed differ from those in the original determination of eligibility?

It is widely recognized that states are out of compliance with the redetermination rules to a considerable extent. Federal regional officials complain about the lack of staff to monitor this situation effectively and more pressing demands for technical assistance and other activities on those staff they do have. The federal government faces several choices with regard to these requirements: increase the surveillance and the penalties for noncompliant states, increase the matching share to encourage states to do a better job, or reduce the requirements so that they are more manageable. None of these options should be exercised in the absence of analyses that demonstrate what the consequences are likely to be in the numbers of eligibles, the use of services, the resulting costs, and administrative feasibility. Moreover, some of the choices, especially those requiring additional funds, will have to be made in the context of other federal priorities and commitments.

The special problems of SSI

SSI eligibility determinations are the responsibility of the Social Security Administration, a federal agency. Applications for benefits under SSI must be taken and processed in much the same way by local federal staff as welfare applications are processed by local welfare offices. In some cases, in fact, SSA has contracted with state agencies for the performance of SSI eligibility determinations.

Two major issues related to Medicaid arise from the SSI process. First, in fifteen states Medicaid eligibility criteria are stricter than SSI criteria. In addition, more than half the states supplement SSI benefits, which further affects Medicaid eligibility (Institute for Medicaid Management, 1978: 23). Thus, Medicaid program staff need to know, not just that applicants are receiving SSI cash benefits, but also the amount of the applicants' income, the value of their additional resources, and other factors that determine their separate eligibility for Medicaid benefits. SSI federalized the former public assistance categories of Aid to the Aged, Blind, and Disabled, but it has not eliminated the need for the states to perform an eligibility determination for supplementation and/or for Medicaid.

Second, even states that cover all SSI recipients for Medicaid benefits need prompt access to a reliable tape of SSI eligibility data in order to verify, sometimes at the point of service and always at claims processing, that a person was eligible for benefits on the day service was rendered. The tapes, however, are frequently late, incomplete, and inaccurate. This is an example of the interorganizational (and, here, intergovernmental) factors that influence the operation of Medicaid. The state's ability to exercise its Medicaid eligibility function depends to some extent on the federal government's ability to supply needed information in a timely manner.[e]

Summary.

Sometimes—perhaps most of the time—a person in need of assistance applies to the public aid department and the system works just as it is supposed to, producing an accurate determination on the question of eligibility in a timely manner. In other cases, however, the system does not do so, thus compounding the hardships faced by people already having trouble making ends meet. The proportion of cases falling into each category is not known, but those in which the system adds to personal difficulties are numerous enough to constitute a substantial problem.

As a formal matter, the processes which produce this situation can be justified only to the extent that they lead to accurate decisions implementing laws and to the extent that they promote equity within each state, if not between all states. As a matter of public policy, too, their accomplishments must be measured against their costs. That is, how much does it cost to arrive at accurate decisions; how

[e] Similar problems sometimes arise even at the same level of government. SSI and Medicaid officials at the federal level are in different organizational units in HHS. Among the states, in some, eligibility is determined by the public assistance department, and the Medicaid program is operated by the health department; in others, although both functions reside in the same department, they are operated by different divisional units. The principal problem is the availability to one of information generated by the other. The problem is exacerbated when benefits vary according to eligibility. In some states, the medically indigent do not receive the same services as the categorically eligible. When information is not freely or promptly transmitted, the eligible individuals' benefits may be jeopardized, subjecting them to an additional burden.

much inaccuracy can be tolerated; and what are the results in terms of benefits awarded and denied? If the decisions are accurate but could be reached with half the information and half the documentation, then it makes sense to simplify the process. If a substantial proportion of eligibility decisions are not accurate and the procedures militate against accuracy for the reasons discussed above, then it makes sense to simplify the process. If eligibility decisions, though accurate, have little impact on aggregate utilization and expenditures, then again it makes sense to simplify the process and to direct administrative efforts elsewhere.

There is reason to believe, on the basis of material presented in previous pages in this chapter, that neither equity nor greater accuracy is well served by the formidable amount of detail found in the present eligibility determination process. Moreover, as noted, the process results in considerable additional hardship to individuals in need. In the following pages, we will examine—first for grant recipients and then for the medically needy—the aggregate impact of changes in the numbers of eligibles on the utilization and cost of services under Medicaid.

THE IMPACT OF ELIGIBILITY CRITERIA

Grant recipients

We have already noted that people become eligible for Medicaid benefits either by qualifying for public assistance cash grants or, in twenty-nine states, by establishing that they are medically needy. Further, we saw that the relationship of eligibility and expenditures is less direct for categorical recipients than for the medically needy since some of the grant recipients do not use medical services whereas all of the medically needy do utilize them. For these reasons, it makes sense to treat grant recipients and the medically needy separately.

Comparing the numbers of eligibles per 100 residents in thirteen states[f] with the numbers of recipients per 100 residents for every even-numbered year over the nine-year period from 1968 through 1976, we found strong correlation coefficients in all four of the categories considered.[g] They ranged from 0.69 for AFDC adults in 1972

[f] The thirteen states are Indiana, Iowa, Nebraska, Texas, California, Massachusetts, New York, Georgia, Oklahoma, Tennessee, Colorado, Maryland, and Pennsylvania. They were selected to reflect differences from state to state in Medicaid program characteristics and differences in the ratio of physican fees under Medicaid to those under Medicare (as a measure of usual and customary fees). Data on program characteristics were measured using the Medicaid Program Index (see Chapter 1).

[g] The category of Aid to the Blind has been omitted since it is such a small and relatively stable category.

Table 4–3. Relationship of Eligibles, Recipients, and Expenditures, Selected States, (Per Capita)[a]

A. Eligibles and Recipients

	1968	1970	1972	1974	1976
Elderly					
Correlation coefficient	.949	.755	.793	.759	.930
N	11	12	12	13	13
Significance	.001	.002	.001	.001	.001
Disabled					
Correlation coefficient	.790	.765	.782	.734	.817
N	11	12	12	13	13
Significance	.002	.002	.001	.002	.001
AFDC Adults					
Correlation coefficient	.920	.747	.686	.893	.807
N	11	12	12	13	13
Significance	.001	.003	.007	.001	.001
AFDC Children					
Correlation coefficient	.810	.909	.857	.829	.877
N	11	12	12	13	13
Significance	.001	.001	.001	.001	.001

B. Eligibles and Expenditures

	1968	1970	1972	1974	1976
Elderly					
Correlation coefficient	.518	.570	.692	.561	.580
N	11	12	12	13	13
Significance	.051	.026	.006	.023	.019
Disabled					
Correlation coefficient	.570	.733	.810	.717	.742
N	11	12	12	13	13
Significance	.034	.003	.001	.003	.002
AFDC Adults					
Correlation coefficient	.853	.806	.342	.838	.815
N	11	12	12	13	13
Significance	.001	.001	.138	.001	.001
AFDC Children					
Correlation coefficient	.828	.842	.736	.706	.828
N	11	12	12	13	13
Significance	.001	.001	.003	.003	.001

C. Recipients and Expenditures

	1968	1970	1972	1974	1976
Elderly					
Correlation coefficient	.563	.713	.607	.502	.630
N	11	12	12	13	13
Significance	.036	.005	.018	.040	.011
Disabled					
Correlation coefficient	.876	.932	.766	.845	.741
N	11	12	12	13	13
Significance	.001	.001	.002	.001	.002
AFDC Adults					
Correlation coefficient	.948	.953	.599	.846	.714
N	11	12	12	13	13
Significance	.001	.001	.020	.001	.003
AFDC Children					
Correlation coefficient	.985	.965	.967	.880	.711
N	11	12	12	13	13
Significance	.001	.001	.001	.001	.003

[a]See Table A–9 for the Medicaid data on which these calculations were based. Note that the number of eligibles are taken from monthly figures for December of each year, whereas the other data are annual figures. Population data was taken from the U.S. Bureau of the Census, *Statistical Abstract of the United States* for the years indicated. The number of states varies because of missing data.

to 0.95 for the elderly in 1968. All of the resulting twenty coefficients were significant at the 0.02 level, moreover (see Table 4–3A).

The relationship between the number of eligibles per 100 residents and the rate of expenditures in those same states was also quite strong, though somewhat less so for the elderly, and, even for them, the relationship was substantial. Excluding AFDC adults in 1972, the range was from 0.52 to 0.84, and all but one of the coefficients were significant at the 0.05 level or less (see Table 4–3B). In sixteen of twenty instances, the relationship between eligibles and recipients was somewhat stronger than the relationship between eligibles and expenditures. None of these results is very surprising—it is to be expected that the number of recipients will increase if the number of eligibles increases and that the amount of money spent will increase if eligibles and recipients increase—but the magnitude of the correlation coefficients is striking.

When we shift our efforts to try to explain *changes* in the per capita numbers of eligibles and recipients and the rate of expenditures, the relationships are somewhat less clear. When 1968 figures are compared with those for 1976, the relationships between eligibles and recipients and between eligibles and expenditures are more variable (see Table A–10 for correlation coefficients). These results occur partly because in 1968 some states were still operating under the old medical vendor payments provisions of the Social Security Act and had not yet adopted a Title XIX (Medicaid) program. These programs were, in some instances, quite different from the programs later adopted under the new title. In addition, the fact that this was particularly true for one of the thirteen states in our sample (Tennessee) means that that single state assumes a disproportionate influence in the calculations.

We employed two strategies to cope with these factors. First, we used Spearman's rank-order correlation coefficient to measure the relationship since it treats each state as the equal of every other state and does not give disproportionate weight to the case that skewed the distribution. Table 4–4 shows the results. The relationship between eligibles and recipients is distributed widely, from 0.555 for the elderly to 0.891 for AFDC children. The relationship between eligibles and expenditures ranges between 0.655 and 0.909. The sign was negative for the elderly reflecting the fact that SSI added the largest numbers of recipients in states with the most limited benefits. Second, we compared 1976 with 1970 instead of 1968. The correlation coefficients (see Table A–11) as well as the Spearman rank-order coefficient (see Table 4–5) were generally weaker and in a somewhat narrower range. The relationship of eligibles and recipients ranged from 0.547 to 0.620 for three of the four categories, and

Table 4-4. Changes in Eligibles, Recipients, and Expenditures, Selected States, (Per Capita) 1968-1976[a]

Spearman Correlations

	Elderly	Disabled	AFDC Adults	AFDC Children
Eligibles/Recipients				
Corelation coefficient	.555	.873	.827	.891
N	11	11	11	11
Significance	.038	.001	.001	.001
Eligibles/Expenditures				
Correlation coefficient	-.655	.909	.682	.800
N	11	11	11	11
Significance	.014	.001	.010	.002
Recipients/Expenditures				
Correlation coefficient	-.227	.836	.564	.845
N	11	11	11	11
Significance	.251	.001	.035	.001

[a]Colorado and Pennsylvania are omitted because 1968 data are incomplete.

the relationships between eligibles and expenditures were between 0.308 and 0.812, except that the coefficient for the elderly was negative. The relationships between recipients and expenditures were substantially weaker and not statistically significant.

These calculations reveal that, while eligibility has a lot to do with the number of recipients and the amount of money spent in a given year, it has considerably less to do with the change over a period of years. The reason for this difference may be that state officials and providers alike focus largely on financial considerations in making decisions. A major goal for public officials is to contain increases in expenditures, but, since the states cannot control them directly, they take other actions, like tightening eligibility criteria, which are intended to influence expenditures by reducing the numbers of people for whom the state will finance the use of medical services. The number of eligibles fluctuates, as well, with ups and downs in economic conditions; they increase as the economy worsens and decrease when it improves.

In part to compensate for the loss of revenue resulting from reductions in the number of eligibles, some providers may raise rates or increase the number of services provided to recipients. Finally,

Table 4–5. Changes in Eligibles, Recipients, and Expenditures, Selected States, (Per Capita) 1970–1976[a]

Spearman Correlations

	Elderly	Disabled	AFDC Adults	AFDC Children
Eligibles/Recipients				
Corelation coefficient	.741	.636	.804	.762
N	12	12	12	12
Significance	.003	.013	.001	.002
Eligibles/Expenditures				
Correlation coefficient	-.469	.727	.811	.636
N	12	12	12	12
Significance	.062	.004	.001	.013
Recipients/Expenditures				
Correlation coefficient	-.063	.182	.692	.308
N	12	12	12	12
Significance	.423	.286	.006	.165

[a]Massachusetts is omitted because 1970 data were not available.

since inflation causes the same service to cost more one year than it did the previous one, even with stability in the number of eligibles and in utilization rates continuing increases in expenditures would be observed.

Restrictions in eligibility criteria have some impact on utilization and on expenditures. But while the effects of such policies on Medicaid expenditures for grant recipients are not insubstantial, they are achieved at the cost of excluding people in need from the program's benefits. For this reason, therefore, their potential in reducing Medicaid expenditures further is limited. We turn now to a consideration of eligibility and the medically needy.

The Medically Needy

As noted earlier, Title XIX offered the states federal financial assistance for part of the cost of medical care for people who, although they met other criteria for public assistance, had incomes somewhat higher than those allowed for grant recipients. The 1967 Amendments to the Social Security Act limited the amount of the income differential to 133.33 percent of the maximum amount paid to an AFDC family of comparable size. Twenty-nine of the fifty states plus the District of Columbia have taken advantage of this provision in the federal law.[h] By so doing, they automatically increase their financial liability under Medicaid; since the people who qualify under these provisions would not have become eligible under public assistance provisions, the state's potential responsibility for medical bills is increased.[i] Thus one way for states to limit their Medicaid expenditures is to have no provisions for the medically needy.

Of those states that do cover the medically needy, however, it must be asked, how much difference does the point at which they set their eligibility standard make? If they make it harder to become eligible for benefits, will they reduce their financial exposure even though they have programs? These questions can be answered in part by comparing the medically needy eligibility level (the Medically Needy Protected Income level, MNPI) with the appropriate public assistance eligibility level. When these two figures are plotted on a graph for those states that include the medically needy, the resulting differences can be described as the "medically needy band," a curve of varying widths and signs.

Given the ostensible purposes of the medically needy category, one would expect that states that included them would have a band located above the public assistance eligibility level since the medically needy are assumed to have more income than public assistance recipients but not enough to meet their medical bills. Thus, for example, if AFDC benefits were payable in a given state to families of four with incomes of less than $3,600, it might be expected that similar families with incomes of between $3,600 and $4,800 would be eligible for medical benefits, with the exact level established by state regulations.[j] It turns out, however, that a number of states have *negative* medically needy bands because their medically needy protected income levels are actually *below* those of the public assistance eligibility levels. Recent figures show that ten of the twenty-nine states with programs had negative bands for AFDC children in 1974, and nineteen of twenty-nine had negative bands for the elderly (Davidson, 1979).

By almost every measure, a negative medically needy band saves a state money. The number of medically needy children as a proportion of all children in a state, the amount of the medically needy expenditure per child in the state, and the amount of the medically

[h] Arizona has no program.

[i] The relationship is not perfect, however, since some people may become eligible for public assistance cash grants because large medical bills have impoverished them.

[j] In the example, if $3,600 is also the maximum amount paid to AFDC families of four in the state, then $4,800 (133.33 percent of $3,600) is the maximum MNPI for families of four. Families with incomes above $4,800 can also become eligible by incurring medical expenses which effectively reduce their income to that level. This process is known as "spending down."

Table 4–6. Effects of Medically Needy Protected Income Level for AFDC Children, 1974[a]

	Medically Needy Children as Percent of All Children	Medically Needy Expenditures per Child in the State (in $)	Medically Needy Expenditures per Child Recipient (in $)
Positive Medically Needy Band (19 states)			
Range	0.5–8.4	0.77–28.69	96.34–783.36
Median	2.2	6.93	247.59
Mean	2.5	8.64	345.23
Negative Medically Needy Band (10 states)			
Range	0.1–3.8	0.22–11.14	91.75–427.00
Median	0.9	0.59	191.69
Mean	1.1	2.55	219.34

[a]See appendix Table A–12 for the data on which this summary is based.

needy expenditure per recipient are all lower in states with negative bands than they are in states with positive bands (see Table 4–6).

Since grant recipients were almost 90 percent of those who used services under AFDC provisions in 1974, however, and since they accounted for almost 85 percent of AFDC-related Medicaid expenditures, the total financial impact was relatively small. Moreover, medically needy recipients and expenditures have declined in importance for AFDC-related Medicaid expenditures still further since then.

For the elderly, the medically needy band produces mixed results (Table 4–7). In those states in which Medicaid eligibility is automatic with SSI eligibility, a slightly higher mean proportion of elderly residents used services as medically needy (9 percent as opposed to 5 percent) in states with a positive band than in states with a negative band. Moreover, expenditures per elderly state resident were somewhat higher in states with positive bands. Excluding New York, whose costs are much higher than those of any other state, the mean expenditure was $170.26 as opposed to $147.71. But, even with New York included, the median expenditure per elderly recipient was almost $800 less in states with a positive band than the comparable figure for states with negative bands. (When New York is excluded, the mean expenditure per elderly recipient, too, is less than in states with a positive band.) The differ-

Table 4–7. Effects of Medically Needy Protected Income Level for the Elderly, 1976

	Medically Needy as Percent of All Elderly Residents in State	Medically Needy Expenditures per Elderly Resident in State (in $)	Medically Needy Expenditures per Elderly Recipient (in $)
Automatic States			
Pos. Med. Needy Band			
(7 states)			
Range	0.052–0.207	$92.70–$526.77	$1,344.08–$6,333.54
Median	0.064	185.03	1,889.38
Mean	0.092	221.19	2,641.42
Neg. Med. Needy Band			
(12 states)			
Range	0.013–0.089	$60.39–$241.46	$1,332.61–$3,851.17
Median	0.047	146.18	2,759.62
Mean	0.052	147.71	2,531.32
All States (19 states)			
Range	0.013–0.207	$60.39–$526.77	$1,332.67–$6,333.54
Median	0.057	146.29	2,629.11
Mean	0.067	176.29	2,574.14
209 (B) States			
Pos. Med. Needy Band			
(3 states)			
Range	0.081–0.088	$186.12–$271.70	$2,117.13–$3,358.53
Median	0.083	240.70	2,888.40
Mean	0.084	232.84	2,788.02
Neg. Med. Needy Band			
(7 states)			
Range	0.018–0.066	$43.71–$237.10	$1,797.79–$3,912.15
Median	0.043	101.22	2,206.00
Mean	0.047	113.02	2,387.04
All States (10 states)			
Range	0.018–0.088	$43.71–$271.70	$1,797.79–$3,912.15
Median	0.062	20.67	2,337.84
Mean	0.083	148.97	2,507.33

Source: Appendix Table A–13.

ences in expenditures are somewhat larger and more consistent in the states that apply a more restricted standard in determining eligibility for the medically needy elderly. Since only two states have positive bands, however, and a third has no band at all, the results must be considered unreliable.

The proportion of the elderly receiving benefits is actually slightly higher in states using a more restricted standard than in the states in which Medicaid eligibility is automatic with SSI, and average expenditures are only slightly lower ($27 per resident and $67 per recipient). Moreover, when New York is excluded, the mean expenditure per elderly resident in the automatic states is less than $7 higher than in the 209(B) states, and the mean expenditure is almost $96 less.

Thus the negative medically needy band apparently saves a state some money on the elderly, but not very much, especially in those states in which eligibility is automatic with SSI. Furthermore, the effect of the more restricted standard is negated by the requirement that all of the elderly in those states be permitted to establish eligibility by spending down, which virtually eliminates the income criterion for eligibility.

To obtain a more complete picture of the dollar effect of both the medically needy band and the more restricted standard, we would need to figure in the cost of living in the states and to calculate estimates of the total dollars represented by the respective options, which is beyond the scope of this work. Short of that, however, the data already available suggest that the results achieved by applying a more restricted standard do not justify—at least on cost-containment grounds—the considerable administrative effort needed to implement it, not to mention the increased hardship it places on families to qualify for benefits.

CONCLUSION

Making it harder to become eligible for Medicaid benefits apparently reduces Medicaid utilization and expenditures. For people who also receive cash grants, however, much of the increase in expenditures remains to be explained by other factors. Having a component for the medically needy and pegging eligibility criteria higher than those for cash assistance logically increases the financial exposure of the state. Some states have attempted to reduce that exposure by using more stringent eligibility criteria for the medically needy than for the categorically needy. That strategy has produced little overall impact, however, since the medically needy are a small proportion of the program for children and since the differences are insubstantial for elderly SSI recipients. Further, restricting Medicaid eligibility for SSI recipients apparently has little impact because of the spend-down requirements.

In the next chapter we turn to a consideraton of the impact of the scope of services on utilization and expenditures.

Benefits

5

Title XIX of the Social Security Act, as amended, requires that all state Medicaid plans include the following basic services: physician services, outpatient and inpatient hospital services, nursing home services, lab and X-ray services, early and periodic screening, diagnosis, and treatment (EPSDT) services for children, family planning services, home health services, and transportation to and from the site of covered services. Beyond these, the federal law specifies a list of optional services for which federal financial assistance is available that includes virtually any other health care service imaginable. Within those broad limits, the states have two basic decisions to make: (1) which, if any, of the optional services to cover; and (2) how much of any covered service to pay for. Thus, a state may decide to cover (or not to cover) services provided by optometrists and podiatrists and to pay (or not to pay) for prescription drugs. It may also decide that, even though physician services must be included, it will pay for only ten visits in a year (or only twenty hospital days or one hundred nursing home days). Further, although it chooses to cover prescription drugs, an optional service, it may only pay for a maximum of three per month and impose a 50-cent copayment fee on each one. Each state may decide to limit services in such ways, or it may decide to impose no limits.

The justification for limitations is that they act as a rationing device. Eligible recipients will exercise care in using services, so the thinking goes, for fear of exhausting their allowable benefits. Further, providers will not furnish more services than are covered for fear of not being paid. Moreover, nonessential services may be excluded altogether on the grounds that the public is ethically or morally required to provide for poor people only those services that they absolutely need. Those other services can wait, some argue, until eligibles become economically self-sufficient or choose to spend their own money on them. In all cases, it is expected that the result for the state will be lower expenditures.

These arguments are countered by those who contend that restricting the range of covered benefits skews utilization in the direction of inappropriate services, which may also be more expensive than the more appropriate services for which they are substituted. To take an extreme example, in a state that did not cover prescription drugs except as part of the cost of a hospitalization, a patient might be hospitalized just so that the necessary drugs could be provided. Or a patient in need of an eye refraction might go to an ophthalmologist, since physician services are covered, instead of to an optometrist, even though the latter could perform the service equally well at less expense.[a]

There has, to date, been no systematic evidence to resolve this controversy, or even to determine the extent to which variations in covered services affect the amounts spent by various state Medicaid programs. We will attempt a partial answer, at least to the latter half of the question, after discussing the extent of the variation among the states.

STATE VARIATIONS IN COVERED SERVICES

Title XIX permits state Medicaid plans to include a broad list of services:

1. Inpatient hospital services.
2. Outpatient hospital services.
3. Other laboratory and X-ray services.
4. Skilled nursing facility (SNF) services (other than in an institution for tuberculosis or mental diseases) for individuals twenty-one or older.
5. Physicians' services rendered in the office, patient's home, hospital, skilled nursing facility, or elsewhere.
6. Early and periodic screening, diagnosis, and treatment of physical and mental defects for individuals under twenty-one (EPSDT).
7. Family planning services.

---

[a] The same effect might occur when appropriate providers, while not excluded from participation by the scope of the benefit package, are nonetheless discouraged from participating by other state policies. For example, if office-based physicians do not choose to see Medicaid patients, poor people in need of services may seek them in a more expensive hospital emergency room.

8. Medical care, or any other type of remedial care recognized under state law, furnished by licensed practitioners within the scope of their practice as defined by state law (such as podiatrists, chiropractors).
9. Home health care services.
10. Private duty nursing services.
11. Clinic services.
12. Dental services.
13. Physical therapy and related services.
14. Prescribed drugs, dentures, and prosthetic devices, as well as eyeglasses prescribed by a physician skilled in diseases of the eye or an optometrist, whichever the patient may select.
15. Other diagnostic, screening, preventive, and rehabilitative services.
16. Inpatient hospital services and skilled nursing home services for individuals aged sixty-five and over in an institution for tuberculosis or mental diseases.
17. Intermediate care facility (ICF) services.
18. Inpatient psychiatric hospital services for individuals under twenty-one.
19. Any other medical care and any other type of remedial care recognized under state law and specified by the Secretary of the Department of Health and Human Services, such as Christian Science nurses' services and skilled nursing home services for individuals under twenty-one (Commerce Clearing House, 6231).

Title XIX, as originally passed, required that at least the first five services be provided to Medicaid recipients. To that extent, therefore, there has been a common minimum benefit package from the beginning. The amounts and duration of those services and coverage of optional services, however, have varied considerably among the states. The law was changed in 1967 to say that if the state Medicaid plan includes the medically needy it must make available to them either the first seven services or any other seven services listed. However, if the plan includes inpatient hospital or skilled nursing facility services for the medically needy, it must also include physicians' services when they are administered to patients in hospitals or SNFs, even if physicians' services are not otherwise covered for them (45 CFR 249.10 [1] [1]–[2]).

Amendments have resulted in the following additional requirements.

Table 5-1. Optional Services Covered by State Medicaid Programs, 1975

	1 Group Covered for Basic Services[a]	2 Optometrist	3 Podiatrist	4 Chiropractor	5 Clinic	6 Dental	7 Physical Therapy	8 Eye Glasses	9 Prescription Drugs	10 Prosthetic Devices	11 Other Diagnostic, Screening, Preventive, Rehabilitation	12 Inpatient Hospital for Elderly in T.B. Hospital	13 Inpatient Hospital for Elderly in Mental Institute	14 Intermediate Care	15 Inpatient Psychiatric for under 21 Years Old.	16 Emergency Hospital Services	17 Private Duty Nursing	18 Skilled Nursing for under 21 Years Old
Alabama	×	×						×	×	×		×		×	×	×		×
Alaska	×														×	×		
Arkansas	○	○	○	×	×		○	○	×	×		×	×	×	×	×		×
California	×	○	×	○	○	○	○	○	○	○	○	○	○	×	○	○		○
Colorado	○	○	×			○	×	○	×	×	○		×	○	×	×		×
Connecticut	○	○	○	○	○	○	○	○	○	○			○	○	○		○	○
Delaware	×	×	×		×		×	×	○	○	○	×	×	×		×		
D.C.	○	○	○		○		○	○	×	×	○	○	○	×	○			○
Florida	×	○			×	×		○	×	×	×	×	×	×		○		×
Georgia	×	×	×		×	×		×	×	×		×	×	×		×	×	○
Guam	○	○			○	○	○	○	○	○						○		○
Hawaii	○	○			○	○	○	○	○		○	○	○	×		○		×
Idaho	×	×	×	×	×	×	×	×	×	×	○	○	×	×		×		○
Illinois	○	○	○	○	○	○	○	○	○	○	×			○		○	○	×
Indiana	×	×	×	×	×	×	×	×	×	×	×	○	×	×		×	×	○
Iowa	×	×	○	×	×	○	○	○	×	×		○	○	×	○	○		×
Kansas	○	○	○	○	○	○	○	○	○	○	×	○	○	○	○	○		×
Kentucky	○				○	○	○	○	○	○	○	○	×	○	×	○		×
Louisiana	×	○	○	○	×	○	○	○	×	×	○	×	○	×	○	×		×
Maine	○	○	○	○	○	○	○	○	○	○		○	○	○		○		○
Maryland	○	○	○	○	○	○	○	○	○	○	○	○	○	○		○	○	○
Massachusetts	○	○	○	○	○	○	○	○	○	○	○	○	○	○		○	○	○
Michigan	○	×	○	○	○	○	○	○	○	○	○	×	○	○	○	○		○
Minnesota	○	○	○	○	○	○	○	○	○	○		○	○	○	○	○		○
Mississippi	×	×			×	×		×	×			×	×	×		×		×
Missouri	×	×			○	○		○	×			×	×			○		○
Montana	○	○	○			○	○	○	○	○		○	○	○	○	○	○	○

Nebraska	o	o	o	o	o	o	o	o	o	o	o	o	o	o	o	o	o
Nevada	x	x	x	x	x	x	x	x	x	x	x	x	x	x	x	x	x
New Hampshire	o	o	o	o	o	o	o	o	o	o	o		o	x	o	x	o	x
New Jersey	x	x	x	x	x	x	x	x	x	x	x	x	x	x	x		o	x
New Mexico	x	x	x	x	x	x	x	x	x	x	x		x	x	o	x	x	x
New York	o	o	o	o	o	o	o	o	o	o	o	o	o	o	o	o	o	o
North Carolina	o	o	o	o	o	o	o	o	o	o	o	o	o	o	o		o	o
North Dakota	o	o	o	o	o	o	o	o	o	o	o	o	o	o	x	o	o	x
Ohio	x	x	x	x	x	x	x	x	x	x	x	x	x	x	o	o	x	
Oklahoma	o	o	o	o	o	o	o	o	o	o	o		o	o	x		o	x
Oregon	x	x	x	x	x	x	x	x	x	x	x	x	x	x	x	x	x	x
Pennsylvania	o	x	o	o	o	o	o	o	x	o	x	o	o	o	o		o	o
Puerto Rico	o		o	o	o		o		o	o	o			o				
Rhode Island	o	o	o	o	o	o	o	o	o	o	o	o	o	x		x		x
South Carolina	x	x	x	x	x	x	x	x	x	x	x	x	x	x	x	x	x	x
South Dakota	x	x	x	o	o	x	x	x	o	o	o		x	o		x	o	o
Tennessee	o		o		o	o	o	o	x	o	o	o	o	o		o		
Texas	x	x	x	x	x	x	x	x	x	x	x	x	x	x	o	o	x	
Utah	o	o	o	o	o	o	o	o	o	o			o	o	o	o		o
Vermont			o	o	o		o	o	o	o			o	o	o	o		o
Virgin Islands																		
Virginia	o	o	o	o	o	o	o	o	o	o	o	o	o	o	o	o	o	o
Washington	o	o	o	o	o	o	o	o	o	o	o	o	o	o	o	o	o	o
West Virginia	o	o	o	o	o	o	o	o	o	o	o	o	o	o	o	o	o	o
Wisconsin	o	x	o	o	o	o	o	x	o	x	o	o	o	o	o	o	o	o
Wyoming	x		x		x		x		x		x		x	x		x		x
Summary:	x=21 o=32	x=18 o=24	x=15 o=24	x=11 o=18	x=13 o=28	x=16 o=29	x=12 o=24	x=15 o=26	x=21 o=29	x=17 o=25	x=9 o=16	x=13 o=20	x=16 o=24	x=24 o=25	x=10 o=16	x=19 o=24	x=6 o=15	x=16 o=26

Key: x = Service offered to categorically needy

    o = Service is offered to categorically and medically needy

SOURCE: Commerce Clearing House, Medicare–Medicaid Guide, State Plans, June 1975.

[a]The basic services include inpatient and outpatient hospital services, physician's services, skilled nursing facility services, laboratory and x-ray services, early and periodic screening, diagnosis and treatment services for children (EPSDT), and family planning services.

1. Provisions must be made for insuring transportation of recipients to and from providers of services, and the state plan must describe the methods that will be used (45 CFR 249.10 [1] [5] [ii]).
2. Early and periodic screening, diagnosis, and treatment services (EPSDT) must be provided for eligible individuals under twenty-one (45 CFR 249.10 [a] [3] [iv]).
3. Family planning services must be provided for qualified individuals (Social Security Act, Section 1905 [a] [4] [c]).
4. A state plan must include home health services for any eligible individual who, under the plan, is entitled to skilled nursing facility services (45 CFR 249.10 [a] [4]).

It is evident, then, that a state's decision to include or exclude a service from its Medicaid plan is another form of variation that affects the comprehensiveness and uniformity of the services available to Medicaid eligibles. Table 5–1 summarizes state decisions in this area. As indicated in the first column, all states cover the nine basic services currently required under federal law for the categorically needy. Next to each state named, beneath the heading "Basic Services," a "o" indicates those states in which all of the basic services required for the categorical eligibles are available to the medically needy as well (thirty-two states). Columns 2 through 18 of the table indicate the states' decisions regarding the inclusion of optional services in their Medicaid plans. A state may choose (1) to exclude a service, (2) to cover the service only for the categorically needy, or (3) to cover the service for both the categorically needy and medically needy. The final rows of columns 2 through 18 indicate the number of states that elect each of these choices for each optional service.

The great variability in state decisions makes the table difficult to summarize, but examination of several services reveals the following:

Optometrists' Services (column 2)
Not covered in eleven of the fifty-three plans.
Covered for the categorically needy only in eighteen plans.
Covered for the categorically needy and the medically needy in twenty four plans.
Dental Services (column 6)
Not covered in eight of the fifty-three plans.
Covered for the categorically needy only in sixteen plans.
Covered for the categorically needy and the medically needy in twenty-nine plans.
Physical Therapy and Related Services (column 7)
Not covered in seventeen of the fifty-three plans.
Covered for the categorically needy only in twelve plans.

Covered for the categorically needy and the medically needy in twenty-four plans.
Prescription Drugs (column 9)
Not covered in three plans.
Covered for the categorically needy only in twenty-one plans.
Covered for the categorically and the medically needy in twenty-nine plans.
Intermediate Care Facilities (column 14)
Not covered in four plans.
Covered for the categorically needy only in twenty-four plans.
Covered for the categorically needy and the medically needy in twenty-five plans.

Table 5-2. Number of Optional Services Included in the State Plans, by State, 1975

Alabama	9	Montana	15
Alaska	5	Nebraska	15
Arizona	no program	Nevada	16
Arkansas	10	New Hampshire	14
California	16	New Jersey	16
Colorado	9	New Mexico	12
Connecticut	15	New York	17
Delaware	7	North Carolina	13
D.C.	14	North Dakota	16
Florida	9	Ohio	16
Georgia	12	Oklahoma	6
Guam	9	Oregon	17
Hawaii	11	Pennsylvania	14
Idaho	8	Puerto Rico	7
Illinois	16	Rhode Island	8
Indiana	14	South Carolina	15
Iowa	11	South Dakota	12
Kansas	16	Tennessee	8
Kentucky	11	Texas	10
Louisiana	10	Utah	15
Maine	17	Vermont	10
Maryland	13	Virgin Islands	5
Massachusetts	16	Virginia	13
Michigan	16	Washington	16
Minnesota	17	West Virginia	15
Mississippi	7	Wisconsin	16
Missouri	7	Wyoming	3

Table 5–2, by indicating the number of optional services covered in each state plan, captures the same data from another perspective. It can be taken as one measure of program breadth, and it too indicates that the states vary widely. For example, Wyoming covers only three optional services, while New York covers seventeen.

While the preceding discussion of the benefit package in each Medicaid program provides an overview of the variation in state plans, this is at best a superficial picture. Tables similar to these have appeared in many congressional documents and HEW publications (see such tables in Institute for Medicaid Management, 1978). This kind of shorthand, while useful for many purposes, hides the fact that a more subtle form of variation among states occurs *within* the broad framework of whether or not a state covers a service; this variation arises from the particular definition of each covered service used in the states. The Code of Federal Regulations reads:

A state Medicaid plan must specify the amount and/or duration of each item of medical and remedial care and services that will be provided to the categorically needy and to the medically needy, if the plan includes this latter group. Such items must be sufficient in amount, duration, and scope to reasonably achieve their purpose. With respect to the required services for the categorically and medically needy, the state may not arbitrarily deny or reduce the amount, duration, or scope of, such services to an otherwise eligible individual solely because of the diagnosis, type of illness or condition. Appropriate limits may be placed on services based on such criteria as medical necessity or those contained in utilization or medical review procedures. (45 CFR 249.10 [a] [5] [i]

This section permits states to define the parameters of each service included in its Medicaid plan. They do so by imposing limits on the duration or scope of services (such as the number of days of inpatient hospital services within a specified time period) considered reimbursable. In addition, the states may require that the medical necessity of some services by certified *before* they are actually given (i.e., prior authorization) in order to qualify for payment.

The types of limitations imposed by the states vary in their details. While this prevents their being summarized neatly, Table A–14 presents the variations by state for selected services. It demonstrates, for example, that most states do not limit the duration of skilled and intermediate care, although many require prior authorization of their use. In contrast, twenty states do limit the duration of inpatient hospital services to some extent.

Table A–15 provides a more general picture of the restrictions imposed by the states on seven required services. For the original five basic services, the table reveals the following:

Inpatient Hospital Services
Six plans apply both limits and prior authorization.
Twenty-eight plans apply either limits or prior authorization.
Twenty plans apply neither limits nor prior authorization.
Outpatient Hospital Services
One plan applies both limits and prior authorization.
Nineteen plans apply either limits or prior authorization.
Thirty-three plans apply neither limits nor prior authorization.
Laboratory and X-Ray Services
Ten plans apply either limits or prior authorization.
Forty-three plans apply neither limits nor prior authorization.
Skilled Nursing Care (for eligibles over 21 years old)
Five plans apply both limits and prior authorization.
Eighteen plans apply either limits or prior authorization.
Thirty plans apply neither limits nor prior authorization.
Physicians' Services
Two plans apply both limits and prior authorization.
Thirty plans apply either limits or prior authorization.
Twenty-one plans apply neither limits nor prior authorization.

To get a better sense of the nature and extent of these limitations where they exist, it is worth looking at some examples. Table A–15 showed that thirty-four jurisdictions limited inpatient hospital services to some extent. Included among these were South Carolina and Florida, which restricted the reimbursable days a patient can stay in a hospital in a year to forty and forty-five, respectively. To understand the meaning of these limitations, we must take note of the fact that only 3.3 percent of Medicaid patients discharged from general hospitals in FY 1976 had stays of thirty days or more *(Medicaid States Tables, FY 1976*, 1978: Table 46).[b] If we assume that 60 percent of those were hospitalized for forty-five days or less, a reasonable estimate, then the maximum proportion of Medicaid discharges with any uncovered days in that year would be 1.3 percent. Thus these limitations are likely to save very little money on hospital services. Moreover, it is also reasonable to assume that patients who need to stay in a hospital forty or forty-five days are especially ill. These limitations, then, place the resulting financial burden on the

[b] Because of the way the data are presented, it is not possible to determine more exactly the number hospitalized for forty or forty-five days.

shoulders of very sick, very poor people, or on the hospital providing the care (since, on ethical grounds, the hospital cannot discharge the patient who needs to be there, nor can it collect payment for the services rendered).

Several states limit hospital stays not on an annual basis, but for each spell of illness. Thus Kentucky permits stays of only twenty-one days per admission, and Idaho, of twenty days per admission. Since the average length of stay for all Medicaid admissions (regardless of eligibility category, age, or diagnosis) in 1976 was 6.95 days, and since 87.3 percent of patients were discharged before fourteen days elapsed (*Medicaid State Tables, FY 1976*, 1978: Table 46), the same questions posed above can be asked concerning these limits as well. On the one hand, they will affect few recipients for few of their hospital days, thus saving relatively little state money; and, on the other, they will hurt most those patients (and the hospitals in which they are receiving care) who are sickest. On these grounds, Utah's limit of 60 days per spell of illness is even harder to understand. It must affect extremely few patients, and those who are affected must be the least able to bear the burden.

Table A–15 also showed us that thirty-two state plans included limitations on physicians' services. A number of states restricted covered physician visits to twelve per year or one per month. Among these are Colorado, Georgia, and Louisiana. There are no data to show us how many Medicaid patients used more than twelve visits in 1976, but the average number of visits per recipient in that year was only 5.7, ranging from 4.4 for children to 8.9 for disabled adults (*Medicaid State Tables, FY 1976*, 1978: Tables 59–65). Since physician visits are relatively inexpensive, the size of the fiscal benefit to the state from imposing arbitrary limits on the number of visits permitted in a year depends on the number of potential visits not made. How many patients will decide not to go to the doctor out of fear that they will use up their allotment of visits before the end of the year? Since no financial burden is imposed on the patients (perhaps because they would have trouble handling it), they have no economic reason to let such a limit be their guide in using services.

If the fear is that patients will go from physician to physician, it is the physicians who are willing to treat them who will suffer the financial consequences if the visits provided turn out to be above the limit. Since physicians have no way to know whether patients they are treating have exceeded their limits, such a policy on the part of a state may exert its effect on expenditures for physicians' services primarily by discouraging physicians from treating Medicaid patients at all. And, to the extent that this happens, patients needing care will be forced to use hospital emergency departments, whose costs are much higher than those of private physicians. (I will say more about these issues in Chapter 8.) If the states' concern is the unscrupulous entrepreneurs who operate high-volume "Medicaid mills" in inner-city ghettos, undoubtedly more efficient means could be found to deal with them without reducing the ability of sick patients to obtain appropriate care from providers qualified to give it.

Finally, some of the limitations apply differently to the categorically needy (i.e., public assistance recipients) than to the medically needy (see Table 5–1). Nine of the twenty-nine states that include the medically needy do not cover identical services for both groups. Pennsylvania, for example, covers dental services and prescription drugs, among others, only for the categorically needy. Similarly, Michigan covers optometrists' services, and Wisconsin covers optometrists' services, eyeglasses, and prosthetic devices only for the categorically needy. Since it must be assumed that medically needy people also suffer from conditions that would benefit from these services and since, with a Medicaid identification card, they probably assume they are entitled to those services as well as to others, the limitations increase the difficulties for the medically needy in those states. They also add to the burdens faced by providers, who must determine not only whether the patient is eligible for Medicaid benefits, but also the nature of that eligibility. One likely result is that providers affected by these provisions will be discouraged from participating in Medicaid. Since money is saved, at least in the short run, it would be worth knowing the benefits and complete cost of such policies, but unfortunately data to determine them are not yet available.

A final component of the benefits picture concerns the extent to which the states change their covered services.[d] Table A–16 demonstrates the extent to which states changed the number of optional services and the number of limitations on five basic services between 1970 and 1975. Regarding optional services, in 1970 only Wyoming provided fewer than five, while more than half the states provided ten or more, and three of those (Indiana, New Hampshire, and Wisconsin) offered at least fifteen.[e] In 1975, still only one state covered fewer than five optional services, but the number of states offering ten or more optional services increased from thirty-one to thirty-eight, and the number offering fifteen or more increased from three to twenty-two. The clear trend in that period was toward the inclusion of more optional services, though the extent to which limitations

---

[d] For a more complete discussion of this issue, see Davidson, 1978b: 54–70.

[e] Arizona had no program at all in 1970 and still has not implemented the one its state legislature enacted in 1976.

were applied to the added services is not known. It must be pointed out, however, that other changes imposed limitations on covered services. Although the effect of changes on expenditures is not clear, it must be assumed that they increase the burden on providers to keep abreast of them and, to that extent, tend to discourage providers from participating.

Regarding limitations on the original five basic services, two states, Florida and Arkansas, had substantial limitations or prior authorizations in 1970, and nine states had virtually no limitations or prior authorizations. The remaining thirty-eight states had combinations that varied by the service. By 1975, the number of states with no limitations had more than tripled, to thirty, and another nineteen states had few limits, leaving only Hawaii and Kentucky with substantial limitations. Thirty states reduced the limitations on one or more services, sixteen did not change, and only three added more limitations.

In the nine months between October 1, 1975, and July 1, 1976, twenty-six states changed at least one aspect of their coverage. Some of the changes increased benefits; some others reduced them, including the following: physician visits for chronic, stable illnesses outside hospitals were limited to one per month in Alabama; in Arkansas, recipients were limited to three prescriptions per month; Maryland eliminated payment for hospital inpatient medical-social days (i.e., days without a medical justification, but for which no more appropriate level of care is available); Massachusetts eliminated hearing aids for adults; Michigan eliminated occupational and speech therapy; Maryland eliminated custom foot supports and all disposable medical supplies except for ostomy supplies and those for permanent urinary incontinence.

In some cases, moreover, the reductions were only temporary. For example, Michigan eliminated both physical therapy in long-term care facilities and hearing services, and then, less than a year later, restored them. Moreover, it eliminated vision services, including eyeglasses and related services, and later restored them as well, though with some limitations. Florida reduced inpatient hospital days from forty-five to thirty a year in January 1976 and restored the maximum to forty-five days in July; it limited outpatient hospital services to $50 a year without prior authorization and later raised the amount to $100, with exceptions up to $200.

To sum up, the states have taken advantage of their freedom to determine the types and amounts of services covered under their Medicaid programs, with the result that considerable variation can be found among them. This variation provides a natural opportunity to determine the impact of different benefit structures on program expenditures by comparing expenditure levels in states with different benefit characteristics. We turn to that effort now.

THE IMPACT OF BENEFIT PACKAGES ON EXPENDITURES

Table 5–3 presents rankings on four measures, two of which indicate different aspects of a state's benefit package and two of which reflect measures of Medicaid expenditures. If fewer covered optional services meant lower expenditures, we would expect to see high correlation coefficients because states with more restrictive benefit packages would provide fewer services and, hence, spend less money. Similarly, if more limitations and prior authorizations meant lower expenditures, we would again expect to see high correlation coefficients. Indeed, most of the coefficients are reasonably strong, although the relationship between limitations and expenditures per resident of the state is quite low. The rankings also show a moderate though statistically non-significant correlation between the two descriptors of the benefit package, the number of optional services covered and the amount of restrictions on the five basic services. This result shows that the decisions regarding the two characteristics of state benefit packages are made separately and not always consistently.

Of the two benefit measures, we would have expected that the limitations would have had a larger effect since they relate to the five basic services, which not only are included in all state programs but also tend to be the most heavily used services and, in the case of hospital and nursing home services, the most expensive ones. It is reasonable to assume, as a result of this analysis, that the particular benefit decisions represented in these data do not have a substantial impact on state Medicaid expenditures although the extent and stability of that effect varies.[c]

SUMMARY AND IMPLICATIONS

We have seen in this chapter that, as with eligibility, the states show considerable variation in the benefits covered beyond those mandated for all states and in the limitations imposed on the five more important required services. Those differences limited Medicaid expendi-

[c] It may be that the components of the summary measures used here are not equally important in relation to expenditure levels. For example, some of the optional services or some of the limitations on basic services may turn out to have a greater effect in this regard than others. Further, the effect of differences in purchasing power of the dollars represented in Table 5–3 has not been determined.

tures to some degree but not consistently. It appears that, if the states want to contain Medicaid costs, they must continue to look for promising means to do so. In the next chapter we turn to another aspect of the program over which state officials have control, reimbursement methods and procedures.

Table 5–3. State Rankings, Selected Characteristics, Thirteen States, 1975

	Number Optional Services Covered[a]	Limitations & Prior Authorizations, 5 Basic Services[b]	Medicaid Expenditures per State Resident[c]	Medicaid Expenditures per Recipient[c]
Indiana	8.5	12.5	3	10
Iowa	5	7	1	6
Nebraska	10	9.5	4	11
Texas	4	6	5	7
California	11.5	5	11	2
Massachusetts	11.5	9.5	12	12
New York	13	9.5	13	13
Georgia	6	12.5	9	4
Oklahoma	1	2	8	8
Tennessee	2	1	2	1
Colorado	3	9.5	6	9
Maryland	7	3	7	3
Pennsylvania	8.5	4	10	5

Spearman Rank Order correlation coefficients

Number optional services and number limitations:	R=0.43	n.s.
Number optional services and expenditures per resident:	R=0.58	0.02
Number optional services and expenditures per recipient:	R=0.39	n.s.
Limitations and expenditures per resident:	R=0.09	n.s.
Limitations and expenditures per recipient:	R=0.59	0.03

Sources: Columns 1 and 2: Tables 5–2 and A–15.
Columns 3 and 4: Table A–17.
[a]Low ranking means few covered services.
[b]Low ranking means more limitations & prior authorization.
[c]Low ranking means fewer dollars spent per person.

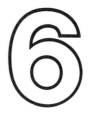

Provider Compensation

Medicaid is a vendor payments program. This means that the state government pays practitioners and organizations providing covered services to eligible beneficiaries so that poor people can receive the health care they need but are unable to purchase out of their own resources. Thus, in addition to determining which people to deem eligible and which services to cover, state Medicaid officials must also make decisions about the payment of providers. Several issues arise here:

1. On what basis should providers be paid?
2. What rates of pay should be used?
3. What procedures should be instituted to pay provider claims?

In this chapter each of these topics is taken up in turn. We examine the choices open to Medicaid officials, the decisions and practices in effect, and the resulting experience.

A fundamental assumption of policymakers considering payment decisions is that provider behavior is affected by those decisions. Thus, if the nature of the responses to the several policy options can be predicted, then policymakers can presumably encourage desired behavior and discourage undesired behavior by their choices. This places two obligations on decisionmakers: first, to know what behavior they want to encourage; second, to know how providers will respond to each option. Neither of these obligations is simple to discharge.

It might be said about the first of those obligations that Medicaid officials want to insure a sufficient supply of accessible services, promote efficiency, and restrain costs—all in a context of an optimal level of utilization of services by poor people—that is, utilization of sufficient services without overuse (see, for example, Holahan et al., 1977). Some decisions promote one good while discouraging another, however, and the formulation lacks operational specificity. Nonetheless, it is worth bearing in mind as we examine particular decisions and the resulting behaviors.

As for the decisionmakers' second obligation, to predict provider behavior is a risky business at best. If the enterprise is viewed from the perspective of open systems theory, it can be anticipated that pressure, in the form of a reimbursement decision, may result in adaptive behavior that cancels the expected gain. For example, a reduction in fees may lead to an increase in the number of services provided. In fact, that very result was observed in Canada under the national health insurance plan in effect there (Marmor, 1975). On the one hand, it can be assumed that physicians will want to maximize their incomes (at least up to a target income) and that they will thus prefer a system that gives them the greatest opportunity to earn what they consider to be enough to satisfy their wants. On the other hand, to the extent that payment decisions influence program expenditure levels, state officials will want to limit physician opportunities to maximize their incomes. The problem is that, although the nature of the opportunities will vary, physicians will have income-maximizing choices—some of which may be harmful to patient health—under any system. The trick is to allow physicians an income they consider sufficient while achieving the goals enunciated above, including the limitation of costs. And the solution may lie in the recognition that the programmatic goal relating to cost is to contain total expenditures, not to limit physician incomes.

I will return to this observation in Chapter 8. First we must take up the question of the basis on which providers should be paid.

THE BASIS FOR PAYING PROVIDERS

Federal regulations regarding payment for providers of services to Medicaid patients cover more than eight double-columned pages in the Code of Federal Regulations (at 42 CFR 450.30). In some cases, those regulations refer to Medicare regulations, which occupy more than ten times that amount of space (at 42 CFR 405.402–405.461). In general, the rules, which vary with the type of provider, aim to establish rates that will insure that high-quality services are available to Medicaid recipients and, at the same time, contain expenditures. In practical terms, the application of these general rules has concentrated more on cost containment than on insuring the availability of services.

Among the major services, payment for hospital inpatient care must be based on the reasonable cost of the service. The regulations state that payment shall be the lesser of the reasonable cost of the service and the customary charges for such services to the general public and that it shall not in any case exceed the reasonable cost payment using the standards and principles developed under Title XVIII, which is Medicare (42 CFR 450.30[1] [2] and [b] [1] and 42 CFR 405.402–405.460). In actual practice, all but ten states (for which the secretary of HEW has approved alternate plans)[a] use the Title XVIII standards for determination of payments for inpatient hospital services.

For individual practitioners, including physicians, dentists, and others, payment is limited to the lowest of the actual charge for the service, the median of the practitioner's charges for that service for the calendar year preceding the start of the current fiscal year, or the reasonable charge recognized under Part B of Title XVIII. In no case can the payment be higher than the seventy-fifth percentile of the range of weighted customary charges locally established under Title XVIII during the calendar year preceding the current fiscal year, the prevailing charge recognized under Part B of Title XVIII in that locality on December 31, 1970, and found acceptable by the Secretary, or the prevailing reasonable charge under Part B of Title XVIII.

It appears that the states, as a result of these rules, have more freedom to establish the basis of compensation for individual practitioners than they do for hospitals. Further, they have used that freedom. As of March 1978, thirteen states used the Medicare method of paying practitioners, eight used a fee schedule either to set the amount of the payment or as a maximum, and twenty-nine used charges with or without setting a maximum. In setting upper limits on the charges to be paid, some states used their own fee schedules and others used the seventy-fifth percentile of prevailing charges (Health Care Financing Administration, 1978: 21). Two observations can be made in summary. First, several states combine methods. Some, for example, base payments on charges but set a maximum established as part of a fee schedule. Second, even after having determined a basis for setting payment rates, states retain considerable discretion in establishing actual rates. For example, they decide when to update the rates regardless of whether they use fee sched-

---

[a] They are California, Colorado, Illinois, Maryland, Michigan, New York, Pennsylvania, Massachusetts, Rhode Island, and Wisconsin. (See Health Care Financing Administration, 1978: 20.)

ules or the practitioners' charges as the basis for setting their rates. (We will return to this issue in the next section.)

For long-term care facilities (skilled nursing facilities or intermediate care facilities), payment must be based on reasonable cost, using methods and standards developed by the state in accordance with cost-finding methods approved and verified by the Secretary. The upper limit is determined by the principles for provider costs under Part A of Title XVIII (which are elaborated in P.L. 92–603, Section 223 and in Title 42 of the Code of Federal Regulations at 405.460–1). In any case payment cannot exceed a facility's customary charges to the general public.

Payment for institutional services was based on costs to ensure that reimbursement levels would rise with the actual cost of the services provided. Thus, it can be argued, the method was designed with an element of fairness in it calculated to win the support and participation of providers. But the method includes no reason for the provider to be efficient or to act to contain costs, perhaps because it was considered easier to audit costs of institutions, many of which already had elaborate accounting procedures in place, than those of practitioners, many of whom practiced individually. It was assumed that charges set by the latter would reflect their costs and that it would be too difficult to attempt to account individually for the costs of each one.

For both institutions and practitioners, therefore, the intent was to pay providers under Medicaid on a basis approaching their payment for services rendered to other patients. In that way, providers would be encouraged to participate, thus ensuring that the low-income Medicaid patient would be able to receive care "in the mainstream" of American medicine.

In the early days, physicians joined the program in part because fees were considered reasonable, with arrangements and even fee levels often negotiated between the state medical societies and administrators of the state programs. Under this approach, however, expenditures for physician services increased to levels that the states considered intolerable. They climbed from $121.6 million in 1965 to $523.3 million in 1969 (Stevens and Stevens, 1974). In response, many states began to limit physician fees, some by instituting fee schedules.

In analyzing 1970 data, Holahan (1975) found that the method of reimbursement affected expenditures for physician services for the disabled, children, and AFDC adults. (He omitted the elderly because much of their care was paid for under Medicare.) He reported that fee schedules reduced expenditures on physician services per user relative to customary charges whether the limit of the latter was the seventy-fifth percentile of fees, as under Medicare, or a lower maximum. He also reported that states using fee schedules to pay physicians had lower inpatient hospital expenditures per use than states using usual and customary fees.

Stevens and Stevens and Holahan, then, were both able to present evidence suggesting that physicians respond to differences in the way they are paid. Stevens and Stevens concentrated on the amount of the fees and their relation to total expenditures for physician services, and Holahan on the methods of payment and their relation to expenditures per user of service. It is clear now, however—perhaps more clear than was possible then—that the focus must be broader. That is, the measure of output must be total expenditures per resident, not expenditures per user of a particular service (because states can vary decisions affecting the numbers of poor who become eligible to use services) or even total expenditures for a single service (because each service is part of a system of services and a reduction in one can lead to an expansion in another). Thus, there has yet to be a comprehensive answer to the question of the effect on Medicaid expenditures of different methods of paying providers.

Before attempting to furnish that more comprehensive answer, we must consider separately the effect of the rates paid to providers. The next section presents data on fees paid to physicians by Medicaid programs and the relation of those fees to the usual and customary fees paid by Medicare. The latter program, it will be recalled, pays physician charges but limits the maximum amount to the seventy-fifth percentile of the prevailing fee for that procedure in the area.

THE RATES OF PAY

Using 1975 data, Burney, Schieber, and their colleagues constructed a ratio of Medicaid fees to Medicare fees. This is of interest because Medicare fees can be taken as approximations of fees paid in the open market for physician services. The amount physicians are paid for a Medicare service is the lowest of the charges they bill, their customary charges for that service, and the prevailing charge in that locality. (The last is defined operationally as the seventy-fifth percentile of the weighted distribution of fees for that service in the area. See Schieber et al., 1976.) The fee indexes were adjusted by a cost-of-living index to attempt to eliminate the effect of practice costs. The ratios calculated by Burney and Schieber (1978) were based on those maximums for twenty-nine procedures as provided by specialists. (The figures can be taken as applying to other physicians, too, however, since although individual fees were usually higher for specialists, the relative fee patterns for general practitioners were similar to

Table 6–1. Relation between Physician Fees under Medicaid and Medicaid Expenditures, 1975

	1	2	3	4	5
State	Average Ratio of Medicaid Fees to Medicare Fees	Medicaid Expenditures per Resident of the State	Medicaid Expenditures perUser of Services	Physician Expenditures under Medicaid per Resident of the State	Physician Expenditures under Medicaid per User of Services
Alabama	100(1)	$36.34(28)	$406.61(40)	$4.54(21)	$50.32(36)
Alaska	100(1)	24.19(46)	851.50(5)	3.71(33)	130.70(1)
Arkansas	92(25)	43.95(20)	505.46(29)	4.16(25)	47.80(41)
California	68(41)	70.38(6)	445.90(36)	11.07(2)	70.11(16)
Colorado	74(37)	38.69(24)	649.21(14)	3.86(31)	64.71(20)
Connecticut	62(45)	52.04(13)	838.93(6)	3.87(30)	62.36(23)
Delaware	100(1)	25.26(44)	298.49(46)	4.53(22)	53.51(34)
D.C.	55(46)	131.43(2)	640.14(17)	19.40(1)	94.51(5)
Florida	68(41)	20.66(48)	447.25(35)	2.25(49)	48.63(39)
Georgia	99(18)	52.02(14)	496.65(30)	7.42(8)	70.79(14)
Hawaii	98(19)	42.72(21)	339.02(44)	6.57(10)	52.15(35)
Idaho	100(1)	29.83(37)	627.18(20)	4.06(27)	85.28(6)
Illinois	79(34)	61.23(10)	426.51(39)	8.44(6)	58.76(27)
Indiana	100(1)	32.47(32)	712.54(9)	2.58(47)	56.67(29)
Iowa	100(1)	28.47(40)	571.32(23)	2.97(42)	59.66(24)
Kansas	87(29)	44.97(19)	657.72(12)	4.67(19)	68.37(17)
Kentucky	100(1)	29.53(38)	280.90(48)	3.79(32)	36.02(47)
Louisiana	89(28)	37.80(25)	360.98(43)	2.82(45)	26.94(50)
Maine	100(1)	57.04(12)	495.14(32)	9.39(4)	81.54(8)
Maryland	52(47)	45.71(18)	469.42(34)	4.28(24)	43.99(44)
Massachusetts	75(36)	84.71(3)	836.77(7)	5.67(15)	55.99(32)
Michigan	87(29)	68.06(7)	652.62(13)	9.88(3)	94.73(4)
Minnesota	100(1)	64.99(9)	1,041.36(1)	4.61(20)	73.92(11)
Mississippi	64(43)	39.96(22)	326.63(45)	6.58(9)	53.75(33)
Missouri	71(38)	20.84(47)	275.79(49)	3.49(39)	46.16(42)
Montana	85(32)	38.90(23)	646.58(16)	5.80(14)	96.49(3)
Nebraska	92(25)	35.10(29)	775.27(8)	2.84(44)	62.74(21)
Nevada	79(34)	27.28(41)	702.13(10)	4.03(28)	103.61(2)
New Hampshire	95(21)	34.46(30)	563.70(24)	4.70(18)	76.00(9)
New Jersey	69(40)	50.08(16)	588.13(22)	5.98(12)	70.17(15)
New Mexico	96(20)	25.25(45)	381.07(42)	3.71(34)	56.03(31)
New York	49(49)	163.06(1)	993.48(2)	8.17(7)	49.77(38)
North Carolina	90(27)	29.95(36)	496.14(31)	3.58(37)	59.33(26)
North Dakota	100(1)	36.95(27)	869.00(3)	2.87(43)	67.52(19)
Ohio	86(31)	34.05(31)	479.44(33)	4.15(26)	58.50(28)
Oklahoma	100(1)	51.86(15)	684.14(15)	5.86(13)	73.28(13)
Oregon	50(48)	32.40(33)	438.70(38)	2.31(48)	31.32(49)
Pennsylvania	39(50)	59.96(11)	532.79(26)	3.64(36)	32.30(48)
Rhode Island	63(44)	77.76(5)	661.28(11)	4.90(17)	41.63(45)
South Carolina	100(1)	26.86(42)	284.56(47)	3.53(38)	37.38(46)
South Dakota	93(24)	31.86(35)	518.07(27)	3.11(40)	50.57(37)
Tennessee	100(1)	29.30(39)	383.44(41)	3.71(35)	48.52(40)
Texas	94(23)	37.64(26)	631.87(19)	4.37(23)	73.39(12)
Utah	100(1)	25.36(43)	546.13(25)	2.77(46)	59.66(25)
Vermont	95(21)	66.42(8)	638.41(18)	8.61(5)	82.76(7)
Virginia	100(1)	32.14(34)	511.62(28)	3.94(29)	62.65(22)
Washington	82(33)	49.68(17)	611.34(21)	6.02(11)	74.08(10)
West Virginia	70(39)	16.04(49)	231.35(50)	3.07(41)	44.30(43)
Wisconsin	100(1)	78.41(4)	862.14(4)	5.12(16)	56.34(30)
Wyoming	100(1)	13.07(50)	444.27(37)	1.99(50)	67.73(18)
Tau_b		−0.071	−0.032	0.0009	0.0564

Sources: Column 1: Ira L. Burney, George J. Schieber, Martha O. Blaxall, and Jon R. Gabel, "Geographic Variations in Physicians' Fees: Payment to Physicians under Medicare and Medicaid," JAMA, 240:13, September 22, 1978, p. 1370. Columns 2-5: Appendix, Table A–18.

Note: Numbers in parentheses indicate state ranking.

those for specialists.) Using their ratio as an indication of the extent to which Medicaid programs pay fees satisfactory to physicians, it is possible to obtain an appreciation of the extent to which Medicaid fees to physicians affect program expenditures.[b]

Table 6–1 presents the average ratios of Medicaid fees to Medicare fees calculated by Burney, Schieber, and their colleagues, as well as per capita state Medicaid expenditures. Using Kendall's tau_b as a measure of rank-order correlation (Blalock, 1972) reveals that the maximum fees payable by Medicaid programs to physicians have virtually no relation to Medicaid expenditures regardless of the expenditure measure used. For total expenditures per resident of the state or per user of services, the statistic shows a negative relationship, which means that the higher the fee, the less is spent on Medicaid. But the relationship is so small that it is practically nonexistent. Moreover, the level of physician fees has an even smaller relationship to expenditures for physician services themselves. But it is worth noting that the two relationships, however small, are in opposite directions. That is, there is a slight positive relation between the fee level and expenditures on services provided by physicians and a slight negative relationship between the fee level and all expenditures. This juxtaposition provides an indication, slim though it is, that it may be possible to decrease total expenditures (or at least contain the rate of increase) while increasing the participation of physicians by raising their fees. While one should be extremely cautious about basing that argument on these data, it is certainly clear that the data show an extremely slight relationship between physician fees and state Medicaid expenditures.

I believe that the primary reason for the absence of a substantial relationship between physician fees under Medicaid and total program expenditures lies in the policymakers' failure to consider that physicians are part of a medical care system and that low rates of pay, which discourage them from providing care to Medicaid patients, result in unnecessarily higher utilization of more expensive substitute services, like those provided in hospital emergency departments.[c] The process of paying physicians, regardless of the rate of pay, may be another reason. If the process is unpredictable, slow, and plagued with errors, physicians who do not depend on Medicaid for

---

[b] Limitations in these ratios are discussed in Burney et al. (1978). They should not be taken as precise, but they are nonetheless reasonable approximations and can be used for the narrow purpose indicated.

[c] It is possible that the extreme weakness of the relationship is also due in part to the fact that the fees used in the analysis were the maximums payable under the various state programs. If the actual fees paid were less than that and the amount of the differential varied across the states, it is possible that the true effect of the fee level was masked.

their livelihoods may choose to avoid the difficulties inherent in the payment system by declining to accept Medicaid patients. (I will have more to say about this subject in the next section.)

Whatever the precise reasons for the lack of relationship between physician fees and Medicaid expenditures, the finding is of particular interest because state Medicaid officials seem so worried about physicians' fees and incomes and have been so reluctant to increase them. The fallacy of this position is that, from a fiscal viewpoint, Medicaid program managers should be more concerned about total Medicaid expenditures than about physician incomes. In the heat of the local political climate, however, the pressures from legislators and others with a limited understanding of the total picture may force program managers to act more quickly and with less attention to the long-term consequences than many would prefer. But it is time now to toss aside the prejudice against physicians that prevails in many state capitals and to redefine the problem to ask, What is the relation of physician participation in Medicaid programs to Medicaid expenditures? In fact, there is logic in the view that *increasing* the participation of primary care physicians, particularly under certain circumstances, is the best way to gain control of Medicaid expenditures (as is argued in Chapter 8). At any rate, the data presented here demonstrate that reducing physician fees, and thereby their participation in the program, certainly is *not* an effective way to reduce Medicaid expenditures.

THE PROCESSING OF CLAIMS

Much of the providers' dissatisfaction with Medicaid arises from the rates of payment used by the programs (see, for example, Garner, Liao, and Sharpe, 1979). But there is another issue of considerable concern: the processing of the claims submitted. There are frequent complaints about delays in payment, inconsistencies in the approval of claims, and the complexity of the forms required. An Illinois study, for example, found that 18 percent of physician claims were rejected on the first pass through the processing system (Illinois Economic and Fiscal Commission, 1976). A similar study, done in Connecticut, reported that 25 percent of bills were rejected the first time they were presented for payment (Connecticut Legislative Program Review and Investigations Committee, 1976). The backlog in 1976, as reported by the Connecticut group, was three months. Another Illinois study showed that, in May 1974, 25 percent of the bills for physicians' and other practitioners' services that were paid by the state's department of public aid were more than four months old and that approximately 5 percent were more than one year old (Davidson, 1974). It takes little imagination to understand that providers with expenses of their own to meet and families to support find it difficult to accept these delays for very long. As one physician wrote, "with the overhead going on minute by minute, and with the pressure from front office staff to see paying patients with problems not requiring this time expenditure, it is a rare physician, in spite of altruism and all other motivation who does not feel reluctant to continually steal time and money from paying patients in order to provide care for more complicated problems of Medicaid [patients]" (see Davidson, 1979).

In order to understand why these problems exist, it is helpful to learn something about how claims are processed. The discussion that follows is based on the Illinois and Connecticut studies already mentioned. It should be taken as indicative of problems found in many states, although the specifics vary from place to place and time to time.

In both of the states studied, processing involves a combination of steps performed by clerks handling paper claims manually, as well as by computers. Typically, a provider submits a claim for payment that includes all or most of the following information: patient name and eligibility or identification number, provider name and identification number, date of service, diagnosis, a description of the service or services rendered, and a price. In many systems, including some that handle hundreds of thousands and even millions of claims a month, bills are sorted by hand according to type of provider, and clerks responsible for particular provider groups then scrutinize them for such things as completeness, legibility, and attachment of applicable prior authorizations (see Figure 6–1, for a summary in graphic form of the process used in Connecticut). Invoices may be rejected at this point for problems in any one of these areas. If a claim passes this review, it is subject to the following steps, some or all of which are performed on a computer:

1. Verification of the client's eligibility for benefits on the date of service. A claim may be rejected if the client's name is misspelled or out of order (that is, first name last, or vice versa, depending on the system), if the number does not match the name, or if the client's eligibility had lapsed or not begun on the date in question. Some of the errors may be corrected by the clerk, perhaps with a phone call to the provider; others result in the claim's being returned to the provider with a notation regarding the reason for rejection.

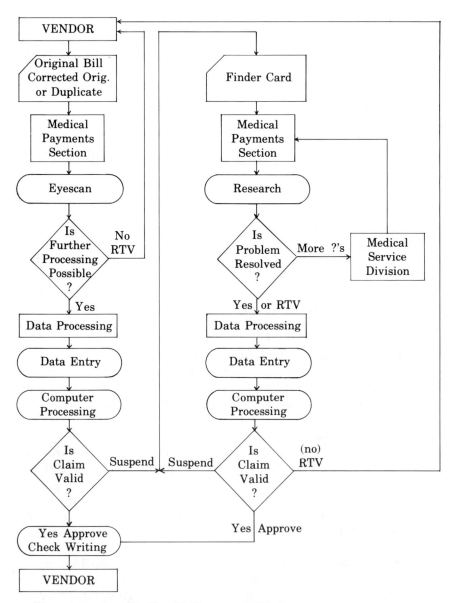

Figure 6—1.   Medicaid Payment System

Source: Connecticut Legislative Program Review and Investigations Committee, 1976:81.

2. Verification of the provider's eligibility to receive payment for the services provided (that is, approved and registered status with the State Agency). A bill may be rejected if the provider is not consid-

ered an appropriate provider of the particular service rendered even if he or she is registered as an approved provider.

3. Determination that an identical claim had not already been filed, processed, and paid. This problem occurs sometimes when the initial claim has remained unpaid for an extended period of time (the exact amount varies with the provider), and the provider has resubmitted it.

4. Determination of whether the recipient of service has other insurance, including Medicare. Medicaid is the payer of last resort and is responsible only for those amounts not paid by other insurers. The extent of this problem is indicated by a study that found that 50 percent of all Title XIX categorical recipients indeed had other insurance (cited in Connecticut Legislative Program Review and Investigations Committee, 1976: 87). Moreover, large numbers of the elderly are eligible for Medicare benefits, and many states "buy in" to Medicare for them—that is, pay premiums, deductibles, and coinsurance (Davidson et al., 1980).

5. Verification that the amount billed does not exceed the amount allowed for the procedure. This is necessary for reasons identified in the section on amount of payment. In addition, in those states that base payment levels on profiles of provider charges, the data must be retained in the computer so the profile can be updated. As indicated above, however, many states are slow and irregular in doing this.

6. Computation of the amount to be paid. Sometimes this is done by hand even in partially automated systems for services that, for one reason or another, have not been coded for computer pricing. In Illinois, for example, at the time of the 1974 report referred to above, burns were hand-priced because of the great variation in the degree of burns, their sites, their extent, and the resulting variations in services needed. It is theoretically possible to precode for the computer almost all services, although to do so would remove some of the system's capacity to respond to unusual events.

7. Preparation of "clean" bills for checkwriting or reports of errors for resolution either by additional manual processing or by returning the claim to the vendor.

The computerized payments system also has the capacity to aggregate the data used to pay claims in ways that permit the monitoring of the system for trends, for fraud and abuse, and for other management purposes. (These functions, which are not really part of the payment system but derive from it, are discussed in greater detail in Chapter 7.)

Several problems associated with claims processing deserve special attention. First is the question of the time that processing takes. It is not surprising that a system with the number of steps listed above requires an extended period to arrive at a paid claim. Clean claims may be paid promptly if the system is an efficient one. It was reported (Davidson, 1974) that Michigan's highly computerized system, which bypasses much hand processing through the use of special forms that can be processed by computer without keypunching by clerks, was able to pay 80 percent of claims within fifteen days and 99.5 percent within thirty days. Further, these results were produced even though the computer rejected 30 percent of claims at the first pass.

In other systems, the elapsed time may be longer, and it varies with the type of provider. The Illinois Economic and Fiscal Commission (1976) reported that the average hospital claim was paid within twenty-six days, and the average physician's bill within forty-one days. The earlier Illinois study showed somewhat higher turnaround times, which varied considerably from month to month and batch to batch. In Connecticut, the department of social services claimed to have paid clean hospital bills within thirty days and all others within forty-five days. The Connecticut Legislative Program Review and Investigations Committee (1976) discovered, however, that only 75 percent of claims were paid "on time," and that 15 percent of those were claims that were "clean" only on the second time around (that is, they had been rejected at least once, but were paid promptly when perfected and resubmitted).

In accounting for delays one report said "the most common reason for rejection of claims is that the computer shows the patient was ineligible at the time of service" (Illinois Economic and Fiscal Commission, 1976: 104). This result may have occurred because the client was in fact ineligible, because the client's identification was entered in error, or because the central eligibility file was not updated promptly. For whatever reason, in many state processing systems such an error will result in the claim's being returned to the provider to be corrected, a step that can add weeks to the time needed to pay what turns out ultimately to be a legitimate claim. In some states the practice is to return claims to the vendor whenever an error is found. In Michigan, this rarely happens because staff try to clean the bill through telephone contact with providers. Still another source of potential delay is the deliberate withholding of payment at various times during the state's fiscal year when the state's cash balance is in danger of reaching unacceptably low points (Illinois Economic and Fiscal Commission, 1976). But whatever the source of delay, it is understandable that providers are discouraged from continuing to treat

Medicaid patients when delays occur in more than a trivial number of cases. Finding ways to reduce imperfect claims and to make the handling of bills, whether clean or not, more efficient will reduce provider frustration and, other things being equal, increase their participation in the program.

Another issue to be raised at this point derives from the fact that such a large proportion of patients have insurance of some kind and that in many states such insurance must cover its share of the claim first. This requires among other things, the timely transfer of relevant data from an insurance company or the Medicare program to the state's Medicaid agency. A report of the National Governors' Conference Task Force on Medicaid Reform (1977) noted that the assignment of benefits under insurance is made to the individual policyholder or the provider of services. That practice places the state's Medicaid agency in the "position of detecting the fact that insurance (or other payor source) exists and initiating administrative action which often costs more than the money collected" (1977: 49). If the existence of other coverage were reliably made known at the time that eligibility for Medicaid benefits were determined, benefits could be assigned to the state at that time. Payments could then be made to the state when it notified the insurer that benefits had been transferred from the provider or recipient to the state, or the Medicaid agency could withhold payment from the provider until payments were received from other insurers. The report concludes that "whatever way is chosen, the essential burden of discovering third-party payors would be removed from the Medicaid program" (1977: 50). Of course, if providers were forced to wait for the competing payors to determine which owed what, they might be further discouraged from participating.

Still another point related to the payment of claims is that, to the extent that pricing is done manually instead of by computer, decisions are made by individual clerks exercising discretion. This practice accounts in part for the unpredictability of payments. Many physicians report that they receive different payments for the same service provided at different times. The greater use of uniform procedure codes would reduce this problem.

States are now required to establish computerized Medicaid Management Information Systems designed by the federal government or equivalent local systems in order to avoid many of the difficulties identified in the preceding pages. States have been slow to take up these systems, however, even though federal funds equal to 90 percent of the development costs and 75 percent of the operating costs are available. There are a number of possible explanations for this reluctance. First, there may be genuine doubt that the expense is worth the potential benefits. Or, perhaps state governments, many of which are headquartered in small cities, do not have the personnel to design or adapt and operate the systems. Moreover, they may be unable to compete for such skilled personnel with higher-paying firms in the private sector. Third, it may be that the state's share of the cost in dollars is too burdensome even though, as a proportion of the total cost, it is modest. Fourth may be that, as the Governors' Conference Report noted, MMIS could result in the rejection of sufficient claims that the states could not meet the thirty-day requirement for processing of claims. A fifth possibility is that these systems do not address patient liability or third-party recoveries (National Governors' Conference, 1977). And finally, the federal capacity to provide technical assistance and approvals for state planning may have been inadequate, at least at earlier stages in the history of MMIS planning (Connecticut Legislative Program and Investigations Committee, 1976; Illinois Economic and Fiscal Commission, 1976). Whatever the reasons, MMIS has not been fully operational in many states, although the number of installations is increasing. As their use becomes more widespread, and as improvements are made, some of the problems discussed above may recede, and the claims payment process may become more predictable and less a deterrent to provider participation in Medicaid programs.

CONCLUSION

In this chapter I have shown that reducing the level of physician fees does not reduce the rate of Medicaid spending. This is true in spite of the fact that low fees apparently do depress the extent of participation in the program by physicians. Inefficient, unpredictable claims payment processes probably contribute to that effect as well. Yet, as noted earlier, once patients enter the medical care system, physicians are the gatekeepers to the utilization of medical services whether they practice in private offices, in prepaid groups, in high-volume inner-city sick-call practices, or in hospital emergency departments. It is pointless to ignore this fact. It would seem, to the contrary, that a more promising strategy to explore, difficult though it may be to bring about, is one that encourages the physician to play his gatekeeping role in the service of cost containment. Before presenting that argument in more detail, however, I will discuss one final method for reducing Medicaid costs—controlling the utilization of services through peer review.

Utilization Control

7

Cost containment through utilization control, the final strategy for containing Medicaid costs to be examined, is predicated on two assumptions: first, a nontrivial amount of the services paid for by Medicaid programs represents misutilization; second, if this misuse is eliminated or substantially reduced, Medicaid expenditures will likewise be reduced. Misutilization falls into three categories: services that are medically unnecessary; services that are inappropriate—that is, although they are justifiable on clinical grounds, they are provided at a level more intense and therefore more expensive than necessary; and services that are considered socially unjustifiable because the cost of the service outweighs the benefit to be gained from it (Stuart, 1977). The attention of Medicaid managers has been focused principally on the first two types of misutilization, although newspapers occasionally report that the admission of a terminally ill cancer patient to a hospital was not certified for Medicaid payment on the grounds that the care was unlikely to produce a cure. These cases raise very difficult ethical issues, and, perhaps because of that, they have not yet become much of an issue in Medicaid administration. Further, when they do arise, the hospital concerned often absorbs the cost of the patient's care, at least in those instances that are publicized. There is evidence, however, that medically unnecessary and inappropriate services do represent problems, although the extent of the problems is less clear.

A variety of studies and reports, some rigorously scientific and others anecdotal or journalistic, has given rise to the assumption that an unknown proportion of the medical care provided to Americans is either medically unnecessary or inappropriate. To the extent that either occurs, medical care expenditures are higher than they need to be. In the discussion that follows, several points should be kept in mind. First, the evidence cited is not limited to Medicaid programs but derives from the American medical care scene in general. The prevalence of the practices may be more or less common under Medicaid, therefore, than is reported generally. Second, while it is undeniable that these practices exist, it is extremely difficult to determine how common they are and how their incidence is distributed among social classes, types of providers, and payment modes. If they are uncommon, or if their occurrence, while not trivial in the aggregate, is widely dispersed, the cost of a serious monitoring and control program might be greater than the potential gain in expenditures saved or recovered. Third, the issue of medical necessity is an extremely difficult one to pinpoint because, as we saw in Chapter 3, much of medical practice depends on the judgment of the professional, not on a tested formula, and well-trained, competent physicians usually have a variety of choices in treating patients who present with a given set of symptoms. Fourth, some misutilization probably does not originate with the providers but results from pressures put on them by patients who want them to "do something" for their problem. In fact, in many instances patients attempt to tell physicians *which* treatment to provide. This is not to deny that physicians are ultimately responsible for their own actions. Rather, it is meant to indicate that, in some cases, they act not out of personal conviction or with an eye to personal gain, but because they are unable to resist the pressure applied by patients who, after all, can take their business elsewhere if a given physician refuses to comply with their wishes. Fifth, some instances of providing care in an inappropriate, expensive site occur because a more appropriate site is unavailable. This may happen in a number of ways—when there are no outpatient facilities for the minor surgery required, when a patient remains hospitalized because no nursing home beds are available or accessible (as, for example, when the proprietor refuses Medicaid patients), or when home health services do not exist in the local area. In such cases, even if misutilization can be established using objective criteria, no satisfactory options are available to the patient or the physician. Finally, monitoring programs whose goal is cost containment must themselves be cost effective; they must not be more expensive than the savings that can be realized from them. (The last point must be qualified, however, to the extent that some monitoring activities serve purposes in addition to cost containment.)

EVIDENCE OF MISUTILIZATION

Misutilization of the kinds indicated above can be inferred from numerous studies. The discussion that follows is not intended to be comprehensive but rather to indicate that there is in fact reason to believe that substantial amounts of misutilization occur.

It is very likely, for example, that a substantial amount of unnecessary surgery is performed in this country. That conclusion is supported by several types of studies. Bunker (1970) found surgeon/population ratios in the United States which were twice as large as those in England and Wales, and rates of surgery two or more times as great here as in the United Kingdom. He concluded that the much higher U.S. rates for many surgical procedures are less likely to be attributable to such large differences in the incidence of the conditions the procedures are intended to correct than to nonmedical factors that encourage the training of more surgeons who, naturally, perform more surgery, at least in the aggregate. Vayda (1973), comparing surgery in Canada with that in England and Wales, found similar results. This strengthens Bunker's conclusion since Canada, although it has a national health insurance program, has patterns of medical practice more like those in the United States than those in the United Kingdom.

Even within the United States, wide variations in the use of surgery depend in part at least on surgeon-to-population ratios, particularly when the surgery is elective and other modes of treatment may be equally effective. Thus Wennberg noted that "studies in Kansas, Vermont, and across Canadian provinces show that overall supply of surgeons and hospital beds strongly affect[s] the incidence rates of surgery (1975: 6). In one of these studies, the likelihood of having certain organs surgically removed was calculated for Vermont, a small state with a relatively homogeneous population, using three years of data (1969 to 1971). It was found that "for the tonsil, the probability of removal by age 26 ranges from 8 percent to 62 percent across thirteen Vermont health planning districts; and by age 75, the probability of loss of uterus ranges from 24 percent to 52 percent." Variations in probabilities of two to three times were also found for removal of appendixes and gallbladders. (It should be pointed out that when data from these studies were reported widely in Vermont, the feedback caused the incidence of tonsillectomies to drop dramatically.) Since differences of this magnitude among residents of a single small state cannot be attributed to differences in the incidence of the clinical conditions among the local population, the conclusion is inescapable that a substantial number of the surgical procedures need not have been performed.

This view is supported by another set of data from studies on the effects of second opinions regarding the advisability of surgery. In New York City, several unions established programs to make a free second opinion available to their members for whom surgery had been recommended. In some cases, the member was required to have the second opinion in order to qualify for benefits under the union's insurance plan; in others, the member had the opportunity to request a second opinion but was not required to do so. McCarthy and Widmer (1974) reported that approximately 24 percent of all procedures recommended were not confirmed by the second opinions and that an additional 2 percent were confirmed but did not require hospitalization. The proportion of cases not confirmed varied with the type of surgical specialty. The authors estimated that the savings from those foregoing the unconfirmed surgery was approximately eight times the cost of the program. The results from this study leave a number of questions unanswered and should, therefore, be regarded as tentative or preliminary. (A study designed to provide more definitive answers is now under way sponsored by the Health Care Financing Administration.) Nonetheless, one is certainly justified in believing that some amount of unnecessary surgery is being performed in the United States.

One of the reasons for the unnecessary surgery, as indicated by Bunker, Vayda, Wennberg, and others, is the oversupply of surgeons in this country. And another result of that oversupply is, in some places, a level of professional activity only half of that judged to be "a full, yet not overburdening, workload" (Hughes, 1975: 184). Hughes and his colleagues compared the activities of surgeons practicing in a suburban community to those in a prepaid group practice with a lower surgeon-to-population ratio. They found that the average surgeon in the suburban community studied spent approximately thirty-six hours in professional activities (the total increased to forty-two hours when time spent on certain professionally related personal activities was added) over a seven-day period. By contrast, surgeons in the prepaid group practice had a total working week of 62.9 hours. Moreover, Hughes reported that the proportion of more complicated or serious operations was higher in the prepaid group practice than in the suburban community and that the particularly difficult operations were usually performed by the most highly trained members of the group. The implication is that, in order to do enough surgical procedures to earn an acceptable living, surgeons in the suburban community performed minor operations, many of which were probably unnecessary, and did not have sufficiently challenging experience to maintain their skills at a high level. Thus, there may be not only negative cost implications to the overpopulation of surgeons, but negative quality implications as well.

Another finding in the studies reported by Hughes showed that in the prepaid group practice studied, which had a financial incentive to provide only necessary surgery and to perform those procedures in the most efficient manner, ambulatory settings were used much more commonly. Thus "almost one in every four general surgical operations was performed on an ambulatory basis" (1975: 185). In the fee-for-service community setting, outpatient sites were much less commonly used. Decreased inpatient services result not only in reductions in medical care expenditures, but probably also in decreased costs to patients since pre- and postoperative time is reduced.

Other research also indicates inappropriate utilization of hospital services. Appropriateness is defined, in these cases, in terms of the site of care. That is, a patient should be in a hospital on a particular day if his or her clinical condition demands the resources and capabilities of a hospital and would not be adequately served by resources available at another level (e.g., in a physician's office, a nursing home, or the patient's own home). Using somewhat different methodologies, Bucher, Gertman, and Rabin (1972) and Zimmer (1974) studied the appropriateness of particular hospitalized days for series of patients in large urban teaching hospitals. Both studies found that 10 to 13 percent of patient days were inappropriately spent in the hospital; and both found that much of the misutilization occurred during short stays and in the middle of long stays. The misutilization arose from such things as inefficiencies in the hospital's performance of tests or transmission of test results and the unavailability of alternative services that, in addition to being more appropriate, would have been less expensive to the medical care system. Thus, if the number of inappropriate hospital days can be reduced, cost savings would result.

Evidence to indicate the misutilization of medical services can also be derived from studies that show widely divergent utilization patterns from one part of the country to another. In 1972, for example, an average of 184.1 per 1,000 southern women aged forty-five to sixty-four were hospitalized for reasons other than for the delivery of a child, compared to 132.5 of 1,000 women from the Northeast; but the latter stayed an average of eleven days, while the former stayed only 8.4 days (Blanken, 1976: 24). More data are needed to understand the full meaning of these figures, but for our purposes they are sufficient to indicate that the patterns of hospitalization in the two areas vary substantially. Women in the two regions are either hospitalized for different reasons, or, if for the same reasons, they are treated using different therapeutic regimens. While they do not by themselves demonstrate misutilization, these data do suggest that patterns of hospital use can be altered to some unknown degree by public policies without harm to the health of patients.

In summary, while it is difficult to estimate precisely the amount, it is reasonable to assume that some of the medical care services provided in this country are the result of misutilization, either because they are unnecessary to begin with or because, although necessary, they are not provided in the most appropriate site of care. Medicaid patients are undoubtedly affected by this situation, but it cannot be said at this time whether their experience represents more or less misutilization than that reported in the studies cited. In fact, there is some evidence to suggest that Medicaid experience is similar to that of other patients (Davidson, 1977). It is also clear that most of the causes for this misutilization lie outside the Medicaid program itself, that they can be found in the presence of too many of certain kinds of physicians, too many hospital beds, and too few less intense services like home health or nursing home services. Nonetheless, it is not unreasonable to believe that reviewing specific instances of utilization or patterns of services may reduce misutilization. In the next two sections, I examine the two principal utilization review methods currently in use: peer review in the form of Professional Standards Review Organizations (PSROs) and medical audit in the form of claims review.

UTILIZATION REVIEW: PSRO

Professional Standards Review Organizations (PSROs) are required in each of 203 PSRO areas designated by the Secretary of Health and Human Services under the 1972 amendments to the Social Security Act (PS 92–603). These organizations of physicians are charged with monitoring and controlling medical care paid for under provisions of the Social Security Act (i.e., Medicare, Medicaid, and Maternal and Child Health Services). The stated purpose of these activities is to "promote the effective, efficient, and economical delivery of health care services of proper quality" (section 2262). PSROs are federally financed by the Social Security Trust Fund and general revenues, and they are advised by groups of nonphysicians in a pyramidal structure extending from local organizations through the states to the national level.

Widespread agreement exists that, despite the multiple goals of the program, PSROs have concentrated on an effort to reduce costs by "curbing certain types of inappropriate use of health-care resources" (Congressional Budget Office, 1979: 1). In particular, they have focused on assessments of the appropriateness of admissions to and length of stay in short-term general hospitals. They have also attempted to monitor the quality of care in hospitals, and PSRO activities are ultimately intended to expand to other sites of care, including long-term care facilities and physicians' offices.

While PSROs have some flexibility in designing their programs, in practice all have adopted the HHS three-part plan:

1. Concurrent review
2. Medical care evaluations
3. Profile analysis

Concurrent review has constituted most PSRO activity during the first several years of operation. It focuses primarily on hospital services at this point (although it will expand to other services as well). Admissions are reviewed against physician-established criteria for medical necessity; and certified admissions, which are approved for a prescribed initial stay, are reviewed as that period expires to determine the need for continued hospitalization. Medical care evaluations are retrospective reviews to determine whether professionally accepted standards of care were met. As of June 30, 1977, 9,370 medical care evaluation studies had been performed by ninety-three PSROs (Health Care Financing Administration, 1978: 4). Profile analysis is the statistical study of utilization patterns and patterns of care provided. The last, which is similar to the claims-monitoring strategy discussed in the next section, is the least well developed of the PSRO activities to date. Since concurrent review, the most highly implemented phase of PSRO activity, is more related to the cost questions which are of primary concern to us, the focus will be on that method of utilization review.

As noted above, concurrent review consists of two principal components, an admission review and a continued-stay review. Under this program, a "review coordinator" determines whether a hospital admission should be certified, usually within twenty-four hours of admission. In making that judgment, the coordinator, usually a nurse, applies locally developed or adapted diagnosis-specific norms. If the coordinator believes the admission is questionable, it is referred to a physician advisor, who reviews the decision and renders a judgment. If the physician decides that the admission is not certifiable, the patient or the admitting physician may appeal to a local committee (and, if still unsatisfied, to state and national review committees).

Those patients certified for admission are assigned a length of stay based on published norms for people of the same sex, age, and diagnosis. That standard is frequently the fiftieth percentile of stays for people with comparable characteristics. If the patient is still in the hospital a day before the initially approved stay is due to expire, the patient's physician may request an extension. A review is then performed by the coordinator, again using locally developed or adapted criteria, to determine whether the patient's stay should be extended and, if so, for how long. Again, it is the physician advisor who makes the decision to reject an extension request; and, again, appeals are possible. In the case of a denial, at either the admission or extension stage, the patient's eligibility for Medicaid (or Medicare or Title V) funds for that admission is terminated.

Under provisions of the law, local PSROs are allowed to delegate the concurrent review function to the hospitals in their area, and as of June 30, 1977, that responsibility was indeed delegated to 76 percent of hospitals.

In its review of PSRO activities, the Congressional Budget Office (CBO) asked three questions:

1. How effective is the program in reducing hospital utilization?
2. Are the associated savings large enough to justify the program costs?
3. Are the program's net savings large enough to warrant the expectation that PSROs will play a major role in containing health care costs?

Following a careful analysis of existing studies, in which methodology was a major focus of attention, the CBO concluded that PSROs had "brought about a modest decrease in the use of short-stay hospitals by Medicare beneficiaries" (1979: 12). The strongest study from a methodological point of view was HCFA's 1978 PSRO evaluation which found "an aggregate reduction in days of care of 1.5 percent" (Health Care Financing Administration, 1978: 178). If that reduction in days of care were applied equally to all PSROs in the HCFA study, the resulting benefit/cost ratio would be 0.892, far short of the 1.7 needed to break even. Moreover, the HCFA report concludes that, even if all of the PSROs were brought up at least to the average impact of 1.5 percent, only fifty-two of the ninety-six areas studied (54 percent) would have had benefit/cost ratios of greater than one.

The answers to the CBO's questions must, therefore, be that the program has a small (1.5 percent) average effect on hospital utilization, that the savings do not cover the costs of the program, and that the program results in savings that are "extremely small relative to federal expenditures for acute inpatient care" (1979: 14). Thus, it is fair to say that, based on the results reported to date, PSROs have not demonstrated their value as utilization reducing and, therefore, cost-saving devices. Several qualifications are in order, however.

First, many of the studies were weak enough methodologically to raise considerable question about their results. Since the conclusions are based on the strongest study, however, it is doubtful that refinements would yield a more favorable picture. Second, the HCFA study showed considerable variation among the PSROs assessed. In fact, Brooklyn and Manhattan, two very large areas in terms of Medicaid use, had benefit/cost ratios of 11.9 and 10.7, respectively (HCFA, 1978: 178). Third, the data are derived from Medicare experience only. Medicaid assessments would be more difficult to make because of inadequacies in assembling suitable baseline data. However, the CBO speculates that there is less reason to expect overutilization of hospital services among Medicaid patients than among Medicare patients (1979: 12–13). Fourth, the PSROs in the study were in different stages of development. The results might have been more consistent if the organizations were equally mature. And, finally, even if their value is limited from the standpoint of effecting reductions in hospital utilization, PSROs might be justified on the basis of other benefits. They may have an educative effect on physicians by making them more aware of the cost implications of hospitalization decisions.

But, even allowing for each of these qualifications, one must wonder if the scrutiny of each hospital admission, not to mention all instances of nursing home and ambulatory utilization, is a sensible approach to cost containment. For one thing, the costs of the process are high. In 1977, each review cost $12.80. While that may be a small proportion of the cost of a hospitalization, it does place a greater burden on the program to produce results. Also, if the participation of physicians in Medicaid is a program goal (as I argue in the next chapter it must be), attention must be paid to the physicians' antipathy to having each utilization decision subject to the review of others, expecially when a physician has few Medicaid patients to begin with and the program staff has no specific reason to suspect him of abuse. For these reasons, I believe it makes little sense to invest much effort in improving concurrent review procedures to the point that they can produce results of the magnitude necessary to justify the program, even assuming that the results could be achieved. It is an expensive process and there is little evidence to justify the expectation that substantial cost savings can be effectuated.

RETROSPECTIVE MONITORING OF CLAIMS

The review of claims on a retrospective basis, by contrast, is unobtrusive and efficient, although it has yet to demonstrate its effectiveness in utilization reductions. It is unobtrusive because it relies on the computer analysis, away from the provider's site, of claims submitted for payment. Thus it need not involve the provider directly, unless a particular provider has, through his or her practices, given some cause. That is the source of its efficiency—it focuses on those providers whose patterns of care (not individual cases, for which there may be extenuating circumstances) give some reason to be concerned about their activities and to believe that enforcement efforts would reveal fraud or abuse in amounts large enough to result in considerable dollar recovery.

Briefly, the system works like this. Under the fee-for-service mode which prevails in the United States, providers of service (whether physicians, hospitals, nursing homes, or others) submit to the state Medicaid program for payment bills on which they identify the amount and nature of services and, in most systems, the complaints or diagnoses for which they were intended. Periodically, those claims, which are computerized, are aggregated and analyzed to determine the patterns of care provided. Thus, for example, a physician might have a profile of services showing that he or she provided an average of six office visits a year to patients twenty-five to forty years old. When that rate was compared to the norm of visits for people in that age group, it might be found that he or she exceeded the average by 50 percent. (These figures are hypothetical.) If the computer were programmed to screen physicians whose visit rates exceeded the average by 30 percent, our hypothetical physician's name would be selected for further review. Similar analyses could be conducted for drugs prescribed, tests or X-rays ordered, hospitalizations, length of hospital stay, and other measures of utilization.

Such results, it should be said, would not constitute prima facie evidence of abuse or fraud or poor practice. They would, however, be reason for further scrutiny since they would be derived not from one patient, who may have had legitimate medical or nonmedical reasons to exceed the norms, but from many patients. Thus, such results would constitute a pattern of practice.

Similarly, the resulting scrutiny—which might take the form of an examination of detailed patient data in the physician's office or the hospital record room—need not be an inquisition in which the presumption is guilt. It can instead be a more modest inquiry into patterns of practice in which the physician or hospital would have ample opportunity to present the reasons for the observed patterns of care. Moreover, the on-site study could be done by specially trained medical personnel (perhaps nurses under the direction of physicians) and not police-type "investigators" or untrained, insensitive clerks.

The method is well described by Rosenberg and his colleagues (1976) and by Mesel and Wirtschafter (1976). It is a part of the Medicaid Management Information System (MMIS), which is a recent requirement of the federal government for continued federal funds. As noted in Chapter 6, states have been slow to establish MMISs or their equivalent, although it appears that more and more have been adopting them. A recent count showed that more than half the states now have an approved MMIS or equivalent capability.

Claims review examines utilization directly, but, as indicated above, less obtrusively and more efficiently than concurrent review under PSRO and similar programs. It has two principal values to program administrators. First, it enables them to detect developing trends in utilization which may require some programmatic adjustment. For example, if, over a period of time, visit rates increase at the same time that the number of providers decreases, it may be that physicians with modest Medicaid practices are withdrawing from the program with the result that patients are more often being forced to use hospital emergency rooms. If that eventuality occurred—and it would be entirely detectable through claims review—administrators would be alerted to search for the causes of increased physician dissatisfaction. In doing so, they might discover a link with a new policy requiring additional paperwork and be able to make suitable adjustments. Second, a claims review system can reduce overutilization and, accordingly, costs. A computer program, once debugged and in place, can be run routinely at relatively little expense, and it can identify suspicious patterns of care. The resulting selective review process that would be triggered by such information could be publicized in such a way as to have a deterrent effect on the few abusers and fraudulent practitioners, and it might cause ordinary practitioners to exercise prudent restraint in cases where they know service is of marginal value.

However, while a good system might produce both of these results, there is no reason to expect that the savings would be so large as to make a big dent in the nation's medical bill. (This assumption is probably as good an explanation as any of Medicaid administrators' slowness to institute MMIS. See Chapter 6.) I believe that most decisions made by physicians and other providers can be justified as the exercise of reasonable professional judgment in the face of uncertainty even when the real benefit of the particular services cannot be demonstrated unequivocally. That is, most decisions are matters of discretion; they do not constitute abuse. And, in the absence of incentives to do otherwise, most practitioners may be tempted to err on the side of providing the doubtful service rather than withholding it. Such a result is even more likely when the program pays them less than they want and they compensate by providing more services. These last comments are based on impressions. Unfortunately, no good data are yet available to demonstrate the actual value of claims review systems.

CONCLUSION

In this chapter I have shown that there is reason to believe that a certain amount of utilization—though it cannot yet be measured precisely—is unnecessary and therefore could be eliminated without harm to patients and at some savings to public medical care financing programs. Two measures to reduce overutilization and the resulting expenditures now in use are concurrent review, associated with PSROs, and retrospective claims review, a part of the Medicaid Management Information System. Neither has yet justified its presence on the scene through substantial reductions in overutilization. The former has a sufficiently poor record and so few redeeming virtues that its continued existence is probably not warranted. The latter is a newer, unassessed system with the virtues of being unobtrusive and relatively efficient. Moreover, it has another potential utility besides its untested impact on utilization control—its value to program administrators in identifying patterns of utilization and trends over time.

This discussion concludes the consideration of the mechanisms that have been used to reduce Medicaid expenditures. None is associated with more than moderate success. Eligibility restrictions and some benefit limitations are associated with somewhat lower expenditure rates but at the cost of reducing the program's ability to improve access to medical services for poor people. Moreover, our inability with the data available to control for other factors (e.g., the extent of poverty and the distribution of medical care resources) makes unclear the actual contribution of these restrictive policies to the observed expenditure patterns. One of the clearest findings is the total lack of association between Medicaid expenditures and the rates at which physicians are compensated. Nor have utilization review mechanisms reliably reduced the amount of services provided. It might be argued that expenditures would have risen still higher without the policies described here, but even if that could be demonstrated, it would be small consolation in the face of the actual increases. Expenditures continue to rise at substantial rates. In the final chapter, after a brief summary, I present a proposal that relies on the dynamics of the medical care system to control utilization.

Physician Participation:
A Proposal to Make Care Available and Contain Costs At The Same Time

The original goal of Medicaid was to make care in the mainstream of American medicine—that is, in the private, office-based sector—available to eligible poor people who needed it but could not afford to pay for it. As the program grew rapidly and program expenditures outstripped predictions, the operative goal became to contain costs, even though increases in other public programs contributed more to the states' growing financial burdens. In the process, the original objective was often obscured.

In previous chapters we have seen that decisions aimed at containing Medicaid costs have not succeeded in doing so. Rising costs have not been curbed by limits on eligibility, on benefits covered, or even on fees paid to physicians. Moreover, even if these attempts had succeeded, it would have been at the expense of the original purpose of the legislation.

I believe that these policies have failed because public officials have taken the wrong lesson from the knowledge that the utilization of medical services by patients in the system is influenced to a very great extent by their physicians. This fact seems to have led policymakers to conclude that, since physicians control the use of services and since, under fee-for-service arrangements, they have financial incentives to increase the care provided in order to raise their incomes, public policies and procedures must limit their capacity to increase those incomes. Thus it was made more difficult for clients to become eligible so physicians would have fewer Medicaid patients; services were limited so physicians would have fewer services on which to collect Medicaid fees; and, most directly, the payment system was adjusted—by lowering (or at least not raising) physician fees and by delaying payments to them—to limit the cash physicians drew from the system.

But these strategies failed because policymakers lost sight of the fact that their goal was not to reduce physician incomes but to reduce program expenditures (or limit their rate of increase), of which fees for physician services are only a part. Physicians remain gatekeepers to most medical services, and Medicaid officials have no power to take that role away from them. In fact, since physicians do control the utilization of services to such a great extent, it is more likely that they would respond to restrictions in Medicaid by exercising that control in ways to limit the financial harm they would suffer from those restrictions in policy. For example, if fees were limited, physicians might provide additional discrete services, charging the allowable amount for each one, in order to bring the total intake up to a reasonable level. And, if payment procedures became too burdensome administratively or too unpredictable, those who could afford to do so might reduce their participation in Medicaid, perhaps even to the point of withdrawing altogether. In fact, both of these eventualities have occurred. The result has been that eligible poor people are deprived of needed medical care and those services that they have obtained have more and more been found outside of the mainstream, in hospital emergency departments. And, contrary to the goal, costs have continued to increase, partly because hospital emergency departments are more expensive sites of care than mainstream physician offices.

These are some of the reasons that the strategies chosen to contain Medicaid costs have not succeeded. In order to be more successful, policymakers must draw the correct lesson from available knowledge about how the medical care system operates. It is not that physicians must be hamstrung in the exercise of their function as gatekeepers to medical services. Rather, it is that physicians, in fulfilling that role, must be encouraged to consider the system-wide cost implications of care-giving decisions. This requires, first, that they return to the Medicaid program—they cannot perform if they have withdrawn—and, second, that Medicaid policies cause them to operate in desired ways. The latter approach, which Schultze (1977) calls "the public use of private interest" involves strategies that induce private actors, who naturally pursue their own interests, to serve the generalized public good by making it identical with their private interests.

In this chapter I first discuss the problem of physician participation in Medicaid—that is, the problem of designing policies that reach the goals of service and cost limitation without driving physicians from the program. I then describe a proposal to make public use of the physicians' private interests by paying them in ways that induce desired utilization experience.

PHYSICIAN PARTICIPATION IN MEDICAID[a]

As we have seen, when Title XIX of the Social Security Act became law in 1965 its goals were to make needed medical services accessible to eligible poor people who could not afford to pay for them and to encourage the use of those services in "the mainstream of American medicine." These goals were to be achieved through a greatly expanded and improved system of payments to providers of medical services, including physicians, hospitals, nursing homes, and other practitioners and institutions. To a considerable extent, physicians are the key to the programs' success because they are indeed "the gatekeepers" to most medical services. Yet, there is considerable evidence that growing numbers of physicians have become disaffected by the program and are either limiting their participation in it or withdrawing altogether.

A 1974 study of California physicians revealed that approximately 40 percent had reduced or intended to reduce their Medi-Cal participation (referred to in Garner, Liao, and Sharpe, 1979). Kushman (1977) found, in 1973 and 1974, that the proportion of California physicians making claims for compensation under the state's Medi-Cal program was as low as 56 percent in some areas of the state. The Michigan State Medical Association reported in 1976 that only 68.3 percent of Michigan physicians indicated that they would accept new Medicaid patients, a drop from 83.5 percent in 1973 (Garner, Liao, and Sharpe, 1979). A Mississippi study conducted in 1976–77 found that only 58 percent of office-based physicians in that state earned $2,000 or more from Medicaid (Garner, Liao, and Sharpe, 1979). And, more recently, the president of the Massachusetts Medical Society (1979) estimated that "physician participation in Medicaid during calendar year 1977 fell to 51 percent of the 14,875 physicians licensed in the state."

The figures vary with the state, the year, and the measure of participation (e.g., the number of physicians seeing any Medicaid patients, the number seeing new patients, the number submitting claims for services rendered, the proportion of visits paid for by Medicaid, or the dollars paid to each physician by Medicaid), but the common theme is that physicians are limiting their participation in

[a] The ideas presented in this section represent the fuller development of material contained in a paper called "Medicaid: The Issue of Physician Participation," prepared for inclusion in *Social Work and Health Policy,* edited by Doman Lum, to be published by Haworth Press.

Medicaid programs, and the phenomenon seems to be a national one. One implication of this fact is that the program goal of insuring care in the mainstream of American medicine is being undermined. Another, more controversial one, is that escalating program costs may be partially attributable to the limited participation or withdrawal of substantial numbers of physicians.

When private practitioners withdraw from the program, many patients turn to hospital emergency rooms that furnish care at prices higher than those charged by office-based physicians (Davidson, 1978a). A North Carolina physician related that in a small, rural county in his state "there are five family practitioners . . . and no other primary care doctors. The physicians charge $10 for an office visit. Medicaid pays them $4.80. Because of this, all physicians stopped seeing Medicaid patients last year. Now a few Medicaid patients are seen by nurse practitioners in the county health department, but most go to the Ambulatory Care Unit of [the local] hospital where Medicaid is charged $21.25 per patient visit and pays $17.02 per visit" (Stephen Edwards, M.D., personal communication).

Furthermore, some states have deliberately fostered the use of public health clinics in the provision of EPSDT services to children, instead of private, office-based physicians, one result of which is higher prices (Foltz and Brown, 1975). In Louisiana, for example, it is reported that when the state division of health bills the division of family services for a screening examination, the cost is 25 to 30 percent more than would be charged by private practitioners (Wallace Dunlap, M.D., personal communication). At September 1975 prices, an office-based pediatrician in North Carolina provided the services recommended under the state's EPSDT program for an average per-visit cost 36 percent less than that of the local health department (Stephen Edwards, M.D., personal communication).

The cost of the program depends on several factors: the number of eligibles, the number of services provided, the types of care provided, and the sources of that care. To the extent that one source is not available, others will be substituted, sometimes at higher unit costs. Further, if the care in those substitute sites is episodic or of poor quality, the result may be a need for additional services that would not otherwise have been necessary. These points, while not yet verified with systematically obtained evidence, raise issues that can be studied empirically.[b]

---

[b] That they represent substantial concerns is indicated by the fact that the Health Care Financing Administration (HCFA), the agency charged with responsibility for Medicaid at the federal level, has twice (in 1978 and again in 1979) solicited research proposals on the substitution of hospital outpatient and emergency department services for those provided in private physicians' offices.

The point, for our purposes, is that, apart from the extent to which the program's original goal is being achieved, there is reason at least to wonder whether increasing the participation of office-based physicians, particularly those delivering primary care, would not help to contain medical care costs. Therefore, it is important to understand what factors influence physicians' decisions about participation in Medicaid.

In October 1978, HCFA funded a two-year, thirteen-state study with three goals: (1) to determine the extent of physician participation in Medicaid programs, using several measures of participation; (2) to identify factors associated with participation, some of which may be susceptible to policy intervention; and (3) to investigate the implications of differing rates of participation.[c] The discussion that follows presents findings from the initial phase of that research, which identified some of the factors associated with participation. It derives from a review of the limited literature available and from an informal survey of pediatricians. Since this part of the study was an effort to generate ideas, not to test hypotheses, it can be said with certainty only that these factors are influential with some physicians. I cannot yet comment on their relative strength when compared with one another, on the proportions of physicians affected by them, or on the extent to which their impact is uniform from state to state.

The underlying thesis is that physicians are influenced principally by fiscal considerations and by factors that interfere with their ability to exercise their professional judgment. This does not mean that physicians will participate only if they get the particular fees they want or that they will withdraw if there is *any* attempt to restrict the extent of their discretion in the treatment of patients.[d] But these are things that physicians care about. Accordingly, if an administrative decision or policy diverges enough from their wishes or expectations, or, more likely, if an accumulation of state actions offends them sufficiently, they are likely to reduce or end their participation in the program, other things being equal.

In previous chapters I have compared state programmatic decisions regarding benefits, eligibility, and payment rates with utilization and expenditure rates. The purpose was to determine the effects of state policies on program utilization and expenditures, and it turned out that, with some exceptions, their effects were

[c] The study, which is being performed by the American Academy of Pediatrics, was funded by HCFA grant number 18-P-97159/5.

[d] Nor that they *should* be free to make absolutely any decision they wish. In addition to professional ethics, a physician should be held accountable for the prudent expenditure of public funds.

limited.[e] In this chapter I will examine some of the same decision areas, but now the intent is to learn why physicians restrict their participation in Medicaid. In other words, to what extent do the same programmatic characteristics, which have limited impact on utilization and expenditures, act as impediments to physician participation in Medicaid?

IMPEDIMENTS TO PHYSICIAN PARTICIPATION IN MEDICAID

Benefits

States are required to cover seven basic services in their Medicaid programs:

1. Inpatient hospital services
2. Outpatient hospital services
3. Physician services
4. Laboratory and X-ray services
5. Nursing home services
6. Family planning services
7. Early and Periodic Screening, Diagnosis, and Treatment services for children (EPSDT)

In addition, the states have the option of covering virtually any other health service available, including transportation to and from sites of care and home health services.

Variation enters in several ways: (1) though all states must cover the seven services, each may set a maximum amount for each service (e.g., fifteen hospital days or thirty) and the conditions under which the seven are available; (2) each state may limit its program to those seven services or add almost any other health care service to its list; and (3) from time to time, states, with federal approval, may change certain aspects of their programs. Decisions on these three factors may limit the care received by eligible patients and, equally, the ability of physicians to exercise their best clinical judgment on behalf of their patients.

---

[e] Eligibility apparently had the largest effect; but it must be recalled that state eligibility policies already exclude 41 percent of poor people from Medicaid benefits (Davis and Schoen, 1978:68), and decisions to restrict eligibility more would further undermine the program's ability to achieve its principal goals.

Limitations.[f]   Inpatient hospital services are provided as long as medically necessary or virtually without limitations in some states (e.g., Illinois, Louisiana, Massachusetts), but in other states a variety of restrictions is imposed. For example, prior authorization may be required for all hospital admissions (e.g., California, Maryland), for stays beyond a certain number of days (e.g., twelve days in New Hampshire, fifteen days in Rhode Island), or for admissions for particular conditions (e.g., renal dialysis or kidney transplants in Georgia, all nonemergencies in Hawaii, cosmetic surgery and surgical transplants in North Carolina). Other states simply set a maximum number of days covered (e.g., ten days per admission in Oklahoma and twenty-one days in Oregon; ninety days for each spell of illness in Ohio; twenty days a fiscal year in Tennessee and forty days in South Carolina).

Similarly, physician services are subject to a variety of rules. In Colorado, for example, a person is eligible for twelve home and office calls in a calendar year; in Arkansas, it is eighteen visits; in Ohio, it is ten visits a month. Other states have no limitations (e.g., North Dakota, Texas, Virginia). Moreover, physician visits for immunizations and routine examinations for children who apparently are well, both of which are established aspects of standard pediatric care, are excluded under Medicaid programs in some states (e.g., Kentucky).

One of the seven basic services that must be part of all Medicaid programs is the Early and Periodic Screening, Diagnosis, and Treatment Program (EPSDT) for children. Under its terms states are required, not only to *pay* for the requisite services, but also to see to it that they are *provided*. The underlying assumption of EPSDT is that if health problems are caught early enough—through early and periodic monitoring—appropriate treatment in childhood can prevent more serious problems later on. EPSDT has been beset by problems since its inception (see, for example, Children's Defense Fund, 1977).

One of the areas of difficulty arises from the fact that some state Medicaid programs do not include the services needed to treat some of the conditions uncovered during screening. As the Children's Defense Fund (1977) writes, "states have strongly resisted the expansion of required services in their Medicaid programs." The ability to achieve the special intent of this program is thus reduced by policies that arbitrarily either exclude required services altogether (e.g., speech therapy to correct problems found during a speech evaluation,

---

[f] Data on the characteristics of state Medicaid programs presented in this and subsequent sections were taken from two sources. They are the state-by-state summaries in the *Medicare and Medicaid Reporter,* published by the Commerce Clearing House (Chicago) and the Health Care Financing Administration's revised report called *Data on the Medicaid Program: Eligibility, Services, Expenditures, Fiscal Years 1966—1978* (Medicaid Bureau/HCFA/DHEW, 1978).

treatment for asthma uncovered during screening, prosthetic devices or orthopedic shoes) or establish restrictions that exclude some children who need treatment (e.g., setting the standard for vision problems at 20/50, thus denying corrective glasses to some children who need them; or allowing only one eye exam or only one pair of glasses in a year, even though some vision problems require more frequent examinations and even though active children may be expected to break their glasses occasionally).

A participating provider of health care services must keep informed about these limitations, as well as about changes in them that affect their compensation for treatment of Medicaid patients. The limitations effectively reduce the practitioner's ability to exercise professional discretion in treating patients. Although often justified as cost containment measures, most of the limitations affect relatively small numbers of patients and only limited amounts of their care.[g] Finally, many of the limitations are on inexpensive services used by few people, which means that their impact on the total state Medicaid budget must be small.

While these characteristics of the benefit structure probably reduce to some extent the amount of services delivered, they may not achieve their larger goals and may create new problems. For example, some of the services thereby omitted may be necessary for the optimal treatment of patients, and some of the omissions may result in the use of additional more expensive services later on. While there is no direct evidence on the extent to which such additional results are produced, it is undoubtedly true that they occur in some measure. In addition, it is likely that these features tend to discourage physicians and other professionals from participating in the program and, to that extent, reduce the degree to which the program's goals are achieved (i.e., fewer patients will be served in the mainstream; and if patients are thereby diverted to more expensive sources of care, costs will be increased unnecessarily).

Changes. States may change their benefit coverage with federal approval. In the nine months between October 1, 1975, and July 1, 1976, twenty-six states changed at least one aspect of their coverage. Some of the changes represented increases in benefits, and some were reductions, including the following: physician visits for chronic, stable illnesses outside hospitals were limited to one a month in Alabama; in Arkansas recipients were limited to three

---

[g] Moreover, it is often possible, though tedious, to circumvent the rules. If prior authorization is required, for example, it is frequently possible to write the request for coverage in a way that cannot be denied.

prescriptions a month;[h] Maryland eliminated payment for hospital inpatient medical-social days (i.e., days without a medical justification, but for which no more appropriate level of care is available); 30-cent copayments on drugs were imposed in Kansas and Mississippi, and 50-cent copayment was imposed in South Dakota; Massachusetts eliminated hearing aids for adults; Michigan eliminated occupational and speech therapy; Maryland eliminated custom foot supports and all disposable medical supplies except for ostomy supplies and those for permanent urinary incontinence. In addition, fees were reduced in a number of states: Florida, for example, reduced its EPSDT screening fee from $10 to $6.25; New Hampshire reduced payments to nursing facilities from 95 percent to 90 percent of allowable cost.

In some cases, reductions were only temporary. For example, Michigan eliminated both physical therapy in long-term care facilities and hearing services and, less than a year later, restored them. Moreover, it eliminated vision services, including eyeglasses and related services, and later restored them as well, though with some limitations. Florida reduced inpatient hospital days from forty-five to thirty a year in January 1976 and restored the maximum to forty-five days in July; it limited outpatient hospital services to $50 a year without prior authorization and later raised the amount to $100, with exceptions up to $200. Even some fee reductions were later restored. For example, in Michigan maximum fee screens were reduced by 11 percent for physicians, dentists, and laboratories, were later restored, and still later were reduced by 4 percent. In Vermont, provider fees were cut by 3 percent and four months later were restored.

Eligibility

Eligibility for Medicaid benefits is intimately tied to the American public welfare system. Recipients of federal Supplemental Security Income benefits (aged, blind, and disabled) are eligible for Medicaid in their states, though in some states eligibility is not automatic. Recipients of Aid to Families with Dependent Children, the federal/state income maintenance program, are automatically eligible for Medicaid benefits. In addition, in more than half the states persons who meet all the requirements for SSI or AFDC except that their

---

[h] This is important not only because some patients may need more than three prescriptions in a month, but also because some pharmacies—partly to compensate for low rates of pay—divide a single prescription in order to collect a double fee (many states pay separately for the drug and for filling the prescription). For example, instead of providing the fifty pills ordered by the physician, the pharmacy may claim to have only thirty on hand and require the patient to return later for the other twenty, at which time an additional fee can be collected.

incomes are somewhat higher, are eligible for Medicaid benefits because they qualify as "medically needy."

Public welfare. Most Medicaid eligibility problems arise from the welfare system. Since welfare is an income support system, it is by definition for people whose incomes fall below standards established by the states, and the states determine welfare eligibility on a monthly basis. That is, individuals may receive public assistance in one month, but, if they are able to get temporary part-time work, for example, they may lose their assistance benefits the following month.

Superficially, at least, this may seem reasonable, given the income maintenance intent of the program, but it has implications that reduce a family's ability to leave welfare permanently (these are beyond the scope of this book) and that, in addition, affect certain aspects of the medical care they receive. For example, the on-and-off nature of eligibility reduces the extent to which a patient can establish a relationship with a single "medical home" providing continuous, comprehensive primary care services. During a month of eligibility patients may see physicians for conditions that need to be rechecked in the month following treatment. But when the patients come for their return appointments, they may no longer be eligible for Medicaid benefits, yet still be too poor to pay the physicians' bills directly. While some physicians will continue to treat such patients, others understandably will not.

The situation is a particular problem under EPSDT, a long-term program with multiple phases extending over many years. The diagnostic and treatment follow-up from a single screening examination may take several months. Keeping in mind that such screenings are intended to occur not only early in a child's life but periodically as well, it can be seen that short-term eligibility can reduce the effectiveness of the program. The Children's Defense Fund quoted a South Carolina EPSDT official as saying that "turnover in eligibility of Medicaid recipients is the biggest problem with EPSDT. People become ineligible as many as three times per year. How are we supposed to give them treatment?" (1977: 143).

Congress enacted a provision in the law, effective in January 1974, that required states to extend eligibility for four months to AFDC families who lost it. The Children's Defense Fund found, however, that, while formal state plans have been brought into conformity with the law, actual practice still limits Medicaid eligibility to shorter periods in some states. Furthermore, persons not receiving AFDC benefits are not covered by the provision; and children with chronic conditions who need ongoing care continue to be left without coverage.

In addition to problems of temporary eligibility, another issue concerns the coverage of newborns. Since eligibility for Medicaid is an individual affair, each potential recipient must be identified separately. Thus, even though a child's eligibility depends on his or her family's income and composition, it must be established individually. Some states permit the mother to register the child prior to birth, but others require the eligibility be established by the mother only after the baby has been born and then only by the mother's visit to a public assistance office to complete the necessary forms. The practical effect is that in some states a newborn is not entitled to Medicaid services even though the mother's prenatal care and the baby's delivery *were* covered. Research shows the first month of life to be critical to the survival of the child, yet care is often denied because eligibility has not been established. At a time when state laws require private insurance companies covering other family members to cover a newborn child automatically for the first thirty days of life, it is anomalous that medical care programs paid for directly by those same state governments do not provide similar coverage.

The medically needy. An additional eligibility problem stems from the fact that twenty-nine states provide benefits to medically needy individuals whose incomes are somewhat above those of public assistance recipients. Those states are permitted to offer a different benefit package to the medically needy than they provide to categorical recipients, and some states have exercised that option. As a result, physicians and other providers in those states must be aware not only of the patients' eligibility for Medicaid benefits, but also the precise nature of that eligibility. For example, Pennsylvania pays for prescribed drugs, dental services, prosthetic devices, and podiatrists' services only for financial aid recipients and not for the medically needy, even though other services are available to both groups. In Maine, clinic services, emergency hospital services, and services in intermediate care institutions are available only to categorical recipients, while other services are available to the medically needy as well.

These rules, in addition to those limiting covered services, reduce the clinicians' freedom to provide the care they determined to be needed by their Medicaid patients. In so doing, they increase the burden felt by the provider who is willing to participate in the program.

Compensating Providers

The most direct deterrents to providers are related to compensation. They fall into several categories: the rates of pay, the speed with which claims are paid, the predictability of payment, and the simplicity of the forms and procedures used. The following discussion concerns payment for physician services only, but it has relevance for other providers as well.

Rates of Pay.   The most common complaint about Medicaid is that the states pay providers at low rates. One survey found that 57 percent of responding physicians identified the fee structure as the one aspect of the program they would most like to change ("Is Anybody Happy with Medicaid?" 1978). In another, 63 percent of physicians in a southerern state complained about "low reimbursement" (Garner, Liao, and Sharpe, 1979). While recognizing the importance of other factors, the authors of two more studies attempted to isolate the impact of Medicaid fees on physician participation in the program. Using data from a national survey of physicians, Sloan and his colleagues found that, "holding other factors constant, a statistically significant fee elasticity of Medicaid participation of .70 was found. If the average Medicaid fee schedule in a defined geographic area doubled, the percentage of a physician's practice devoted to Medicaid patients would increase about 70 percent" (Sloan, Cromwell, and Mitchell, 1977). Examining data from California representing experience over a four-year period, Hadley (1978) found remarkably similar results. His analyses "suggest that a 10 percent increase in average revenue per Medicaid patient would increase participation (for the three specialities in the study) by about 7 percent (roughly from .42 to .45) and the number of Medicaid patients per participating physician by about 18 percent (or almost ten patients)."

As noted previously, some states, as well as the District of Columbia, use the Medicare basis for payment—that is, the seventy-fifth percentile of usual, customary, and reasonable charges for a particular service in an area.[i] Others pay physicians on the basis of reasonable or customary charges (but not at the Medicare level) or fee schedules. But whatever the basis for paying physicians, dissatisfaction arises from state practices of setting fees at rates below usual charges and of failing to revise them to compensate for increases in costs.

When New York first established its Medicaid program, it paid professional practitioners on the basis of reasonable charges, but

[i] This practice creates problems in relation to services not used by Medicare recipients. Medicare does not have financial profiles on pediatricians, for example.

shortly afterward the state shifted to a fee schedule that effectively reduced rates paid for service. The result was a decline in utilization of practitioners' services, as planned, but it is not clear how much of the utilization thus eliminated was overutilization and how much was reasonable. Since the late 1960's those fee schedules have not been revised. The result is that a pediatrician practicing in New York receives $12.00 for any visit for a new illness requiring a complete examination and history to diagnose, and $7.20 for a return visit. Moreover, New York State announced that the $12.00 fee could be charged only once in a three-month period for any child regardless of the child's medical condition. As the director of one of New York's county-operated Medicaid programs has written[j]

> virtually all other classes of providers—hospitals, nursing homes, suppliers of drugs, appliances, etc.—are paid on the basis of rates and prices which are influenced by the prevailing cost of doing business. This results in public and private clinics receiving $40-$80 for a clinic visit for the same service which, if given in the private physician's office, is priced in the State Fee Schedule at $12 if it is the first visit to a pediatrician or, if it is a follow-up or routine office visit, at $7.20.[k]

Similar views are expressed in other states, where fees are often lower than those in New York. In Maryland, for example, the rate is $7.00, with no distinction between a new visit and a return visit.

One question that might be asked is, What is wrong with $12 for an office visit? If four are done in an hour, the resulting $48 does not sound bad for an hour's work. Furthermore, the physician may be able to charge private patients more than $12 and thus raise the hourly figure above $48.

Part of the answer concerns the relationship of the gross payment to the cost of operating a modern medical practice. As one Vermont physician has written,

> The overhead in our practice is 64 percent of gross billings and the fee offered by Medicaid is 61 percent of our regular fee. At the same time, our calculations show that the average gross bill of the Medicaid patient for a visit is 7 1/2 percent higher than for a non-Medicaid patient, but the reimbursement is the same (i.e., 61 percent of the fee). The net

[j] This and subsequent quotations from practitioners are taken from letters from pediatricians who were asked to respond to several questions regarding their experience with Medicaid.

[k] It must be understood that the two rates may not be entirely comparable. The physician's fee includes primarily, if not exclusively, the examination of the patient, while the clinic fee may include the costs of laboratory work, X-rays, and a much higher overhead as well. If services provided as a result of a visit to a private physician but billed separately were added to the physician's fee, the true cost of a visit would obviously be higher, though it is likely that it would continue to be considerably less than the clinic fee.

result is that Medicaid reimburses us 57 percent on the average gross billing for a Medicaid patient, which represents a net loss of seven cents on each dollar charged every time we see a Medicaid patient. . . Seeing a Medicaid patient costs us $9.13 in overhead expenses, and we are reimbursed $8.00.

A physician practicing in the state of Washington made a similar statement:

Reimbursement for standard office calls is slightly above the overhead level in those pediatric offices having small staffs. In an office providing more comprehensive service and having a larger support staff, reimbursement will be at less than the overhead level. . . . With the overhead going on minute by minute, and with the pressure from front office staff to see paying patients with problems not requiring this time expenditure, it is a rare physician, in spite of altruism and all other motivation, who does not feel reluctant to continually steal time and money from paying patients in order to provide care for more complicated problems of Medicaid children.

Another part of the answer is related to characteristics of Medicaid patients that distinguish them from other patients, including the amount of services needed. As a Seattle pediatrician wrote,

Medicaid children are far more difficult and time-consuming to care for than other patients because of the following: (a) language barriers; (b) no home phone to receive the doctor's return call; (c) Medicaid parents report most illnesses after office hours, on weekends, and holidays because that is when they are with their children; (d) major communication problems arise because adults other than the parents frequently take Medicaid children to the doctor's office.

This testimony is corroborated by a Baltimore physician who said,

The effort and time required for the care of a Medicaid patient is often greater than that for one's regular practice because of: (a) the tendency for many of the patients to ignore the making and keeping of appointments—they either don't show up, placing an additional burden on the physician for retrieval, or they arrive with four children instead of one for whom the appointment was made; (b) the frequent lack of telephone facilities; (c) the restriction against telephoning prescriptions; (d) the additional and often cumbersome paperwork; (e) the usual delay of the agency in making payment to the physician; (f) the difficulty of securing consultation through the usual channels.

The Vermont physician mentioned earlier indicated that the services provided to Medicaid patients in his practice are more expensive on the average than those provided to other patients because "Medicaid patients actually require a disproportionate amount of time and support services as compared with others." As we saw, however, the program pays at a rate lower even than office overhead. On the other hand, Vermont officials decided that services provided under EPSDT, administered as part of the same Medicaid program, should be compensated at a higher rate—that is, on the basis of usual and customary charges, which "serves to alleviate some of the problem." In Illinois the opposite is true. Practitioners there are paid more to provide a service under Medicaid than to provide the same service under EPSDT.

Low physician fees are meant to save tax dollars, but Chapter 6 demonstrated that they do not in fact have that effect. To the extent that they result either in an increase in the amount of services provided or in the diversion of services to more expensive sites of care, they lead to higher Medicaid expenditures. When private practitioners withdraw from the program, many patients turn to hospital emergency rooms, which furnish care at higher prices than private practitioners (The North Carolina experience cited earlier is one example.)

Other compensation problems.   In addition to low fees, providers complain frequently about delays in payment, its unpredictability, and the complexity of the forms required (see, for example, Garner, Liao, and Sharpe, 1979). A 1974 Illinois study showed that 26 percent of physicians' and other practitioners' bills paid by the state's department of public aid in May of that year were more than four months old and that approximately 5 percent were more than one year old (Davidson, 1974). A more recent study in Connecticut showed that 25 percent of bills submitted were rejected the first time they were presented for payment and that the backlog on old claims was more than three months (Legislative Program Review and Investigations Committee, 1976). The authors wrote that staffing in the Connecticut medical payments section was at such a low level that work on the backlog could only be done on an overtime basis, which further aggravated the state's financial position.

In some states, particularly those that still rely to a considerable extent on hand processing (as opposed to more extensive use of computers), physicians complain that when they submit a bill they do not know whether it will be paid, and, if it is, whether the amount of the payment will be the same as the last similar bill submitted. The computer promises to bring greater reliability as well as improved efficiency to the processing of claims and the management of the complex Medicaid program. It may not completely alleviate dissatisfaction on the part of practitioners, however, if the forms required appear to be too complex, as reports from a number of pediatricians indicate they may be. While the need for accountability is understandable, many practitioners believe that the forms used call for more detail than is necessary.

IMPLICATIONS AND POSSIBILITIES

It appears from the material presented that, regardless of their intent, many of the policies and practices of Medicaid programs have the effect of increasing the burden on participating providers. Since participation is voluntary, providers are likely to withdraw or curtail their participation to the extent that they can afford to do so. The sources cited above provide ample evidence that many physicians have in fact done exactly that.

This tendency, which has been observed throughout the country, is a matter of concern, in part because it reduces the extent to which the goal of providing care to poor people in the mainstream of American medicine can be achieved. In addition, it is more expensive and less efficient not to rely heavily on primary care practitioners.

Discouraging private physicians from participating in Medicaid results in more referrals of patients to emergency departments of hospitals, more nonreferred use of those emergency departments, more use of public health department clinics (especially for EPSDT services), and more use and encouragement of high-volume "sick-call" offices.[1] Yet none of these sites should be encouraged as principal sources of ambulatory medical care. Hospital emergency departments are overstaffed and overequipped to provide the routine first-contact care people need most. Moreover, they are geared to respond to accidents and to discrete episodes of illness, not to offer comprehensive care with a measure of continuity. Health department clinics—which often are understaffed, established for limited purposes, and operated for less than even forty hours a week—are also ill-equipped to provide primary medical care. And the high-volume, storefront sick-call practices found principally in low-income inner-city areas, while perhaps capable of providing primary care, typically render care as episodic as that found in emergency departments. In addition to these reasons, the fact is that the unit costs in each of these sources are

---

While these assertions are supported by considerable anecdotal evidence, there have been no systematic studies that demonstrate the extent to which they affect Medicaid programs in the aggregate.

higher than those found in typical private practices—whether of the solo, small group, or comprehensive clinic variety—as a number of examples provided above affirm. Thus, greater use of private practitioners should reduce Medicaid expenditures because unit costs are lower.

It is clear from the preceding discussion that physicians limit their participation in Medicaid when the program becomes too burdensome. This is not surprising when we stop to consider that physicians are both professionals trained to exercise independent judgment and small businessmen determined to earn a living commensurate with their position and training and sufficient to support their families comfortably. It should be equally clear that any proposal with a hope of increasing the participation of office-based physicians under terms that accomplish the twin goals of making services available to poor people and containing costs must give due regard to both sides of their character. That is, if a plan arbitrarily restricts physicians' ability to exercise their professional judgment or their capacity to meet their financial requirements, it will fail. That is so for two reasons. First, physicians have the option of withdrawing from the plan and limiting their practices to patients who pay by less onerous methods and at more tolerable rates. Second, should they choose to remain in the program, they have the capacity as gatekeepers or captains of medical care teams to find ways around the limitations that frustrate them. That more and more physicians are choosing not to bother with Medicaid should be a warning against such a policy.

The self-defeating policies described above should clearly be abandoned in favor of others that reduce the burdens of participating physicians. Eligibility policies should provide for more stability; the list of covered services should be comprehensive and devoid of arbitrary limits on the amount of each permitted; administrative procedures should be simplified; and, perhaps most important, payment rates should be reasonable, and payment procedures should be efficient and predictable.[m] While all these aspects can increase physician participation in Medicaid, paradoxical as it may appear, it is the payment system that offers the best hope of containing costs.

The search must be for a payment method that permits physicians to retain their professional autonomy, to earn satisfactory incomes, and yet to be influenced by the costs to the program (and ultimately to the medical care system) of particular treatment decisions. The first requirement in the effort to achieve such a plan is to dismiss the

---

[m] For specific recommendations in each of these areas, the reader is referred to S.M. Davidson, "Medicaid: The Question of Physician Participation," in Doman Lum, ed., *Social Work and Health Policy* (New York: Haworth Press, forthcoming).

erroneous and dysfunctional myths of the past. Then, the warlike atmosphere that often obtains between government official and private physician, in which neither trusts nor respects the other, can be replaced by honest bargaining and negotiation.

This discussion has demonstrated that the single most important area for negotiation—though by no means the only one—concerns the rates and processes of paying physicians for the services they provide. Before government staff begin to discuss financing arrangements, however, they need to understand more about how the practicing physician sees the issues and about the financial implication of running an office. Only then will they be able to design a system with a realistic hope of accomplishing the twin goals of paying for care *and* containing program costs, because only then will they understand how the physician views compensation and why.

Before outlining a specific proposal, therefore, I first discuss the operation of the small business that is a medical practice. Then I present material on the principal options for paying physicians. Finally, I offer some suggestions on considerations to take into account when Medicaid officials make policy decisions regarding compensation for physicians.

A Physician's Office

The first point to be made is that one must distinguish between primary care physicians, whose professional activity is centered in their offices, and surgeons and medical specialists, much of whose time is spent in the hospital. A major implication of this difference is that primary care physicians have much higher overheads to cover than surgeons and even than medical subspecialists. The space and resources used by the latter two—including operating rooms, the laboratory tests and X-rays ordered, many of the assistants who aid them—are all provided by the hospital at no charge. In this connection medical specialists are more like surgeons than primary care physicians although their offices may absorb more overhead than the surgeons'. Primary care physicians, in contrast, spend most of their professional lives in their offices. Patients call or come to see them there, and the services they provide are furnished there. The nurses, technicians, receptionists, and clerks are their responsibility. They must purchase their own equipment and supplies. And they must pay these costs out of revenues derived from fees.

The second point is that, even though their expenses are higher, primary care physicians are the lowest paid of all physicians. They work the longest hours and—depending on the size of their practices and the number of their associates—they may need to be available on evenings and weekends more than their higher-paid colleagues.

Yet, the services they provide are paid at lower rates than those of medical specialists and surgeons. Unlike surgeons, who are paid for particular operations, primary care physicians do few discrete procedures, which are priced at considerably higher rates than equivalent amounts of time devoted to primary care. The principal service offered by primary care physicians is defined by the time they spend with their patients. During that time they interview them to learn about the symptoms and history of their complaints, examine them, and after diagnosing the problem, select an appropriate treatment plan. They explain the plan and the need for patient compliance with it (e.g. taking the medicine until the bottle is empty even if the symptoms have gone or avoiding certain foods for a period of time), and they answer questions. Sometimes tests are performed or ordered. In some instances no therapeutic intervention is called for— that is, the condition (e.g., a cold) is self-limiting, not serious, and unresponsive to medication.

How much should one be willing to pay for ten to fifteen minutes of a physician's time during which the primary activities are talk (no matter how purposeful and regardless of the physician's experience and efficiency) and, perhaps, a brief examination after which the decision is that no therapy is indicated? Say, for the sake of argument, the charge for an initial office visit it $20, which is not an uncommon charge these days, though many physicians charge considerably less[o] (and Medicaid programs pay still less). If physicans can schedule four such visits in an hour and spend five hours in their offices each day, their gross incomes for the day would be $400. From that figure, 50 percent should be subtracted for overhead (a reasonable figure for our purposes; in many primary care offices it is higher) (which reduces the amount to $200. If fees for hospital visits (say $10 per hospitalized patient per day) and the markup on some tests[p] are added, the maximum daily net may rise to $250.

These figures obviously vary with the number of hours worked, the time spent with each patient, and the fee charged, and they are also affected by the number of cancellations and no-shows (patients who do not cancel but do not keep appointments; many physicians attempt to compensate for these eventualities by overscheduling patients for a given time period). But, on the whole, we arrive at a net

[o] To simplify the illustration here I have used figures for initial visits only. Blim et al. (1979) report fees for initial and follow- up visits for several specialties. Charges for follow-up visits average 20 to 48 percent less than those for initial visits. Net income obviously depends in part on the mix of initial and follow-up visits.

[p] Many routine tests performed in the physician's own office are included in the visit charge. If he sends out blood samples or urine specimens and pays the lab for analyzing them, he may add a fee on top of the lab's charge. If he sends the patient to the lab, he will have no part in the financial arrangements between the patient and the laboratory.

weekly income of $1,250 and an average annual before-tax net professsional income of $62,500 for fifty weeks of work.

These figures, which have been arrived at inductively using the assumptions indicated, may even be somewhat higher than those actually earned by average primary care physicians. A 1975 study done under contract from the Social Security Administration showed the average net income (defined as earnings after expenses but before taxes) for five specialties. They ranged from $64,600 for obstetricians and gynecologists to $44,800 for general practitioners. The primary care specialties of internal medicine and pediatrics were $53,900 and $50,100, respectively (Thorndike, 1977). Figures for the same year from the AMA's Periodic Survey of Physicians tended to be somewhat lower for most (but not all) specialty groups. Radiologists reported the highest average net incomes, $75,239, in that survey (American Medical Association, 1978).

In sum, when we discuss primary care medicine, we are talking about a labor-intensive service in which few discrete billable procedures (if any) are performed. Since the rates paid for the physician's time and skill are relatively modest, the hours worked to earn the incomes indicated can be quite long. Furthermore, for pediatrics, a primary care specialty in which the office visit is the principal billed service (Blim et al., 1979), there is the additional fact that third-party payments are much less common than they are for other age groups. Well-child care, an important part of pediatric practice, and office-based services for acute illness usually are not covered by insurance. Therefore, the fees charged are paid directly by the child's family for the most part even though the family may have medical insurance for other services. The demand for pediatric care, therefore, is relatively elastic—higher fees mean that less care is sought.

Finally, regardless of the relative value indicated by the fees it generates compared to specialty services, primary care is complex and challenging. Medicine attempts to define ever more precisely serious diseases of different organs and to develop and apply definitive treatments for those conditions. Primary care problems are more common and often appear to be less important, although the sequelae can be quite serious (see the Harvard Child Health Project Task Force, 1977: Chapter 4). The challenge of primary care is to encourage patients to seek early consultation for potentially serious conditions from a physician who has accepted continuing responsibility for the care of the patient and in whom the patient has confidence. Problems seen by primary care physicians often are subtle and require considerable skill to diagnose. The treatment is frequently restraint in one guise or another—avoiding certain foods, avoiding long hours or certain strenuous activities, even avoiding useless medications. Compliance with the physician's recommendations is, therefore, a crucial issue. It is not a matter of correcting a malformation with a surgical procedure, which, though it may be a difficult task technically, is entirely in the control of the surgeon and his or her assistants. It usually is a question of persuading independent individuals in their roles as patients to accept a recommended course of action—which may include discomfort or inconvenience—when they would rather not do so. The challenge is enormous, and the satisfaction of succeeding in it can be commensurately large, but the material rewards are modest, certainly in comparison to those of other physicians.

The point of these few paragraphs is not to evoke sympathy for conscientious primary care physicians, but to create a realistic context in which to consider the important question of compensating physicians for primary care services under public programs. Following a discussion of the compensation alternatives, I employ this context for a consideration of the policy questions faced by public officials.

Methods of Compensating Physicians

Three principal methods of paying physicians are used in the United States:

Fee for service: A payment is received for each service or group of services actually provided. The fee may be set by the physician or by a third party. A fee schedule is a variation in which fees are set by the third party. In the United States, 71 percent of physicians are paid by this means.[a]

Capitation: A payment for an enrolled person or subscriber is made in advance to cover a specified group of services over a specified period of time regardless of the number of services actually provided. Only 1 percent of U.S. physicians are paid by this means.

Salary: A payment is made by an organization to a physician employee for services rendered on behalf of the organization during a specified period. Approximately 28 percent of U.S. physicians are paid in this way.

In the discussion that follows, I focus on the first two of these choices because, even though more than one-fourth of American physicians are salaried, that method is not an option currently available to public financing programs. Further, when I speak of

[a] Estimates pf physicians paid by each method are from Gabel and Redisch (1979).

methods of paying physicians, I mean the payment from the government program directly to a physician when he or she is the principal caregiver, or to an organization or group of physicians when it undertakes to be responsible for the continuing care of patients. In the latter case, the physicians and other personnel actually providing the care may be employees of the organization and may, in fact, be salaried, but that arrangement is not relevant to our concern here.

Fee for service and capitation present contrasting financial incentives to physicians. Under the former, they have an incentive to provide more services, at least up to some target income. The more services they provide, the more fees they generate, and the larger their incomes will be. Under the latter arrangement, the impetus is to provide fewer sevices because the pool of funds from which payments are made—and, therefore, the practitioners' incomes—may be reduced by the amount spent on services. That is, if services are provided, the fund may be reduced by the amount needed to pay for them—for example, nurses' time, tests, drugs, surgery, hospitalization. The fewer the services provided, the more nearly intact the fund remains.

It should be said explicitly at this point—in order to avoid misunderstanding—that physicians are motivated by more than the financial implications inherent in different payment methods. They are influenced by the intellectual challenge of medical practice, by the ethics of their profession, and, like the rest of us, by the satisfaction of doing a job well. Nevertheless, it is also true that, other things being equal, more services are provided when physicians are paid a fee for each service than when they are paid in advance for whatever care may be needed.

In addition to their respective implications for the amount of services rendered, these two methods of payment have other notable characteristics. Under the fee-for-service mode, the physicians' freedom to provide services is constrained in part by what the payment source will pay. If patients pay directly out of their pockets, physicians are constrained by the patients' own assessments of the costs and benefits of the service. This is the case because individuals are likely to exercise restraint at the point at which they consider making their first visits to physicians for given conditions; once they have taken that step, physicians make most of the decisions regarding the services to be used, and patients generally acquiesce. But if the services are covered by government programs or by the patients' insurance plans, physicians are less constrained by financial considerations in deciding whether or not to provide the service since they can expect to be paid. This point must be qualified to take account of the compensation problems discussed earlier, which have caused many physicians to reduce or end their participation in Medicaid.

When patients are covered by third parties (either private insurance or government programs), physicians (or sometimes the patients in the case of private insurance and Medicare) submit a claim indicating that the service was provided and the charge. Previously a legitimate claim was paid by the third party after routine processing. Now, however, before paying the bill, government programs and some insurance plans make independent determinations of whether the service was necessary or not, particularly for elective surgery. Moreover, the rate of payment to physicians is usually less than their charges for services. Depending on the terms of the program and the capacity of the patients, the physicians may attempt to collect the difference between their fees and the third party's payment directly from the patients. (Under provisions of the Medicaid law, however, physicians are limited to whatever the program will pay.)

Capitation is prepayment. The amount the physician receives from the third party does not vary with the services he or she actually provides for a covered patient. Briefly, a plan in which a physician is "at risk" for all services might operate like this: Premiums are paid by or for insured individuals (or people eligible under a government program) into a large fund. From that fund money is taken as needed to administer the plan, to pay for primary care services, and to pay for other covered services. Dollars remaining at the end of the year are profit (or savings) to be divided between the insurance company and the primary care physician under terms which vary with the particular plan.

As a condition of participation, the insured agrees to seek all care from a participating primary care physician of his or her choice. That physician, in turn, agrees to be responsible for the care needed by his or her patients. Out of the general fund, an account is established for each participating physician, (or group of physicians, including HMOs), based on the number of insured people who sign up with him or her and on their age and sex. Out of this account, the primary care physician receives money for primary care services. These payments may come in regular installments or on a fee-for-service basis. The account must also cover the cost of other services needed by enrolled patients, but only when the primary care physician refers the patient for those services (e.g., a specialist or hospital). Since the primary care physicians may receive year-end bonuses reflecting savings on secondary and tertiary care, they have direct financial incentives to limit the amount of referring and hospitalizing they do. If a physician's account runs a deficit, at the end of the year he or she must repay to the general fund a portion—usually small—of the primary care money received during the year.[r]

One resulting feature of these arrangements is that administration can be simplified for both the practitioner and the third party. Payments can be made at regular intervals (e.g., monthly). They need not be tied to a statement from the physician claiming a service was performed for which payment is due. Changes in enrollment—of patients and physicians—and other aspects of the agreement can be made only at specified intervals (e.g., yearly). Further, monitoring of the patterns of care, as necessary a function under capitation as under fee for service, can be accomplished independent of the payment procedures. Physicians can submit simple utilization forms, for example, indicating that specified services were provided, and these can be analyzed to determine rates of utilization and patterns of care. The resulting analyses can serve two purposes: first, they can protect against underservice by physicians trying to maximize their financial gain; and, second, they can be used to revise rates for the coming year based on expected utilization.

In addition to simplifying the administration of third-party financing plans, capitation also has the advantage of affecting all sectors of the acute care system simultaneously. Fee for service, in contrast, emphasizes and exacerbates the fragmentation of the medical care system. Decisions regarding the provision of services are made by practitioners and patients independently, without relation to decisions made by others. Under capitation, however, if the prepayment covers all services, then utilization of the entire spectrum of medical care can be affected. The primary care physician can control, for example, the amount of specialists' services and hospitalization to be paid for by the third party.

Finally, it is worth noting that either method, when used by government as an instrument of policy, can be designed to achieve a variety of public goals. While the two methods have certain distinctive features, each plan takes much of its character from the specific component decisions that, when added together, constitute a particular payment system. Some of these decisions concern the services covered, relationships between primary and specialty care, and the physician's financial risk.

In sum, then, the two principal modes of paying physicians carry with them contrasting features. Each has proponents and detractors. In choosing between them (and leaving aside for the moment the question of their relative acceptability by government officials and

---

[r] A plan similar to the one described here is already in operation in the private sector in Seattle, Washington (see Moore, 1979).

physicians), it is important to recall the principal policy goals of Medicaid:

1. To make available to eligible poor people the medical care they need but are unable to buy.
2. To contain program costs to a reasonable level.

The first goal, as we have seen, requires the participation of physicians, particularly primary care physicians who will provide continuity and furnish directly or arrange for comprehensive services. The second depends to a large extent on the amount by which hospital utilization can be reduced. The questions that face us, therefore, are, What effect can decisions regarding the method of payment have on these twin goals? And what particular decisions are of most importance?

The first goal—increasing physician participation in Medicaid in order to make needed services available to eligible poor people—can theoretically be achieved equally well with either payment plan. In fact, because of its greater familiarity, the fee-for-service method is probably to be preferred. Certainly it would meet less resistance than capitation, an unfamiliar mode with popular associations to socialized medicine in England. The key to its effectiveness in increasing the availability of services is to raise the rates of pay to primary care physicians and to ease their administrative burden. Then physicians would be attracted to the program in greater numbers, and more services would be available. The drawback to the fee-for-service arrangement is that it may also increase program expenditures. It would result in more service and, perhaps, greater expenditures even though some savings would result from reductions in the use of expensive emergency departments as sites for routine care. If fees were raised by equal rates for all physicians, all would have equal reason to increase services to Medicaid patients; they would have no financial cause to exercise restraint. If fees were raised differentially to favor primary care, additional primary care services would, of course, be provided; and, if nothing else were done, the amount of speciality services and hospital utilization would also increase to the extent that previously unmet needs were discovered through the increased primary care provided. Certainly, at the very least, there would be no reduction in the use of those services.[s]

---

[s] Another way to reduce specialists' services is to lower their fees. This method is not to be preferred, however, since primary care physicians in many parts of the country already report difficulty in prevailing upon specialists to accept Medicaid referrals.

Thus, if the policy goal is to accomplish both of Medicaid's stated objectives at once—increased medical care *and* cost containment—it is likely that government planners will want to consider capitation closely. According to the theory of prepayment, holding primary care physicians (or the prepaid group practice/health maintenance organization) at risk for all of a patient's care causes them to exercise prudent restraint in the provision of services, which results in reduced overall utilization by the covered population. The participation of primary care physicians—an instrumental goal—can be encouraged by setting the rates high enough that they will benefit both from the provision of primary care services (even if there is no year-end surplus to share in) and from safeguards that limit their risk of loss. Regarding the latter, the greatest risk is from patients with serious conditions requiring considerable amounts of expensive hospital care. The two ways to limit the primary care physicians' risk from such cases are to restrict their financial responsibility for any one patient to a reasonable, arbitrary figure (e.g., $5,000) and to limit the amount of money they would be required to pay back if their accounts were overspent (e.g., to 5 percent of their primary care payments).

Assuming the primary care physicians' monthly payments for primary care services alone are high enough to encourage their participation, the advantage to government planners of prepayment over fee for service derives from the primary care physicians' exercise of the gatekeeper function for *all* services needed by their patients. The program would pay only for those services that were provided by or authorized by primary care physicians (except in emergencies). Since the primary care physicians would have financial incentives equivalent to shares of surpluses left in their accounts at the end of the year, they would limit the extent to which they referred patients to specialists or hospitalized them. Further, this result would be achieved without government regulation, which is cumbersome, expensive, and ineffective. In essence, government planners would be relying on the dynamics of the medical care system to control the utilization of services and, thereby, program expenditures.

Two potential secondary benefits are worth mentioning. First, prepayment may lead to a more efficient medical care system. Since primary care physicians would be responsible for all care, they would need to arrange coverage for off times. That, in turn, might lead to the gradual formation of more primary care groups and the greater efficiencies they bring. The tendency may extend to the creation of additional multispecialty groups, too, if primary care physicians establish good working relationships with the specialists to whom they send referrals most frequently. Second, capitation affords an opportunity to give more recognition to the greater amount of time needed to treat the "new morbidity" which includes "a range of illnesses and disabilities arising from social, behavioral, and environmental problems" (Harvard Child Health Project Task Force, 1977: 22), and "many of the most pressing and unsolved child health problems—behavioral and mental health problems, teen-age pregnancy, child abuse" (Keniston, et al., 1977: 157). Currently, physicians are usually paid a fee for each itemized service they provide; and it is hard to put a price on the services required to deal with many primary care problems, including the ones just listed. Capitation, thus, might be particularly appropriate for the provision of services to children.

In sum, by altering the financial incentives for primary care physicians, this proposal has the potential of reducing the utilization of sub-specialist services and, particularly, hospitalization in those instances in which the physician has a choice of treatment options. Since hospital utilization consumes a substantial proportion of Medicaid dollars, it is likely that the magnitude of the savings could be important. It is less clear that services provided in long-term care facilities can be affected by this strategy, but that is a matter for further consideration.

The Politics of Payment

If, then, government planners determined they wanted to try capitation because it offered the potential of achieving the two goals of Medicaid at once, how could they gain sufficient acceptance of it to make it a reality? The fact is that, at the present time, prepayment is likely to be resisted not only by physicans, but also by administrators of state Medicaid programs. (It will be noted that I have referred to government "planners" not "administrators." The roles of the two are different and so are their interests.)

I believe, first of all, that capitation need not be a disadvantage to primary care physicians. In fact, it offers some real advantages. The key is in the component decisions that are made, especially concerning the extent of financial risk and the rates of compensation. In planning, government officials must be reminded that primary care physicians are both professionals keenly interested in preserving the opportunity to exercise the professional judgment they were trained for and, as we saw earlier, small businessmen determined to earn livings commensurate with their positions and training and sufficient to support their families comfortably.

The capitation rate must be set high enough to pay for the expected utilization of services, but low enough to limit the rate of increase in total program expenditures to a tolerable level. To accomplish these objectives, the rate should be divided into two parts:

the first for primary care and the second for other services. Further, the primary care amount—which can be paid to primary care physicians in regular monthly installments— should be set at a level high enough to obtain the participation of primary care physicians in greater numbers and to a greater extent than at present. This means that the rate must be set higher than the equivalent of current Medicaid fees and closer to the fees the physicians command from their private patients.[1] The savings will come in expenditures from the second part of the primary care physicians' accounts, the part used to pay for referral and hospital services. Patients will not go directly to specialists or to hospitals; instead they will be sent by their primary care physicans. And the latter will be more selective in referring or hospitalizing patients because their end-of-the-year surpluses may be reduced otherwise.

Since the operative financial incentive here is to withhold service, some physicians might be tempted to withhold needed services as well as marginal ones. Therefore, it would be necessary to monitor the care given and ordered by the primary care physicians not, as with fee for service, to protect against *over*utilization, but to guard against *under*utilization. This could be done relatively easily by asking the physician to submit simple utilization forms for services provided or ordered. (Since specialists and hospitals would be paid on the basis of authorized claims submitted, their claims forms could serve a purpose similar to the primary care physicians' utilization forms.) These could be analyzed by Medicaid staff, and patterns that did not fall in an acceptable range could be subject to further scrutiny by a reasonable peer review system. In designing this aspect of the program, government planners would be well advised to obtain the advice and participation of practicing physicians.

Thus, capitation could have several advantages for primary care physicians, depending on the decisions made to give it its specific character. It could result in reasonable income from the provision of primary care services. It could simplify administrative procedures by divorcing the receipt of primary care income from the submission of claims. It could provide the physicians with maximum freedom to practice their profession subject in most cases only to after-the-fact monitoring of patterns of services provided. And, finally, the accountability function that is an inherent part of all public programs could be accomplished unobstrusively in most cases.[11] The program would

---

[1] If an additional objective were to increase the number of physicians attracted to primary care, the rates could be increased still further (see Gabel and Redisch, 1979).

[11] Physicians would still be subject to pressures from patients wanting specific services. Under the fee-for-service mode, if they were unable to persuade patients that the requested services were unnecessary, they could yield to such demands, provide the services, and collect the additional fees.

depend to a considerable degree on mutual respect between government officials and practicing physicians.

Since captitation would establish incentives which are unfamiliar to most physicians and patients, it is unlikely that the desired new behavior patterns for either group would occur immediately. Rather, it must be expected that they would develop over time as everyone acquired experience with the new system. Further, capitation would create some problems that would need to be overcome before the full potential could be realized.

First, primary care physicians would need to say "no" to patients who come to them demanding specific services which the physicians consider to be unnecessary and to subspecialists whom the patients have visited without referrals. These denials of service requests may create antagonisms, at least until all participants gain experience and new patterns of behavior become established. Moreover, some primary care physicians may need to sharpen their diagnostic skills in order to distinguish between those who really need to be referred and those who do not. Finally, capitation creates the need to protect not only against *patterns* of underservice, but also against *particular* denials of service. Primary care physicians will make honest mistakes, and some patients may want another opinion to confirm the physician's judgment. While undoubtedly it is possible to establish administrative procedures to perform that function efficiently, the cost savings that are possible under capitation will be eroded if they are resorted to in more than a small proportion of cases.

Even with these caveats, capitation remains an idea in which government planners may be able to interest physicians if the issues are considered honestly and physicians are approached with respect. But there remains the question of how to obtain the support of government officials, particularly program administrators and legislators at the state level. A particular idea to be overcome is the ingrained view that each payment of public funds must be tied to a piece of paper showing that a particular service was performed. The suspicion—born of experience in many spheres—that private vendors are out to bilk the public treasury dies hard. It demands a good system of accountability, but it may be possible to persuade those officials that that function does not necessarily require a claim for each service rendered. In fact, as noted, it is possible to monitor patterns of services provided unobtrusively after the fact and to intervene effectively as the need arises with a sound peer review system. Moreover, if the

Under prepayment, in contrast, their financial interests would coincide with their medical judgments in those instances. Suspicious patients might believe they were denied services because of the financial implications for their physicans. The extent to which this scenario actually occurs and the physicians' responses to it can be determined only with experience.

prepayment plan were good enough, participating physicians would want to protect its integrity and ensure its success and, to that end, would support a strong monitoring system.

The strongest argument for public officials may be that prepayment offers the best and cheapest means of accomplishing both goals of the Medicaid program. Not only would it make primary care and other medical services more readily available to eligible poor people, but it would also contain Medicaid expenditures. Further, it would accomplish these goals with a greatly simplified administration, thus saving additional public funds.[v] It appears, then, that a prepayment plan could serve the interests of both primary care physicians and state Medicaid officials, although both might resist the idea at first. A number of questions remain, however.

For one thing, since specialists and hospitals would continue to be paid for specific services they provided, procedures would be needed to tie them into the prepayment aspect of the program. For example, if they were to be paid only when a service was authorized by a primary care physician, mechanisms to facilitate their obtaining that authorization and communicating it to the state payment agency would be needed. Further, rates would have to be established for them as well. A related question may not be answerable until after the program is in operation. Since the principal savings would result from reductions in the amount of specialist and hospital services provided, what response would the affected specialists and hospitals have? Would specialists raise their fees to compensate for lost business or spend some of their time as prepaid primary care physicians? Would hospitals raise their charges or convert space to other purposes? Another question to be answered is how to get more services to areas that now have insufficient medical care resources. The plan does not deal with this question directly, although an indirect effect of a successful program may be to encourage more primary care physicians to locate in underserved areas, particularly in inner cities. If Medicaid becomes a stable source of reasonable payments, physicians who live in the suburbs of large cities may be induced to work in their centers. Years would pass, however, before such a result could be measured unless specific plans were made to test it on a limited demonstration basis.

Because of these and other questions, which, for the time being, must remain unanswered, the most sensible policy is to experiment with capitation arrangements on a small scale in limited areas and

[v] It should be recognized, however, that streamlined adminstration might result in fewer public jobs and thus create conflicting pressures for legislators. For, while they want to save state dollars, they also need jobs with which to reward the faithful.

for limited periods of time to determine where the bugs are and whether they can be worked out. Moreover, successful demonstrations could serve the additional purpose of helping to persuade interested physicians and program administrators that this is an innovation with potential for solving problems of concern to both.

CONCLUSION

Medicaid and other public programs that rely on the private sector have applied various regulatory mechanisms to achieve program goals and contain program expenditures. In the best of circumstances, such programs pose a formidable challenge to the ingenuity of government planners and policymakers. The sad fact is, however, that the "command and control" approach to regulation (Schultze, 1977), which is typical of such efforts, has failed dismally. Moreover, it is particularly inappropriate in the decentralized medical care sector, which has large numbers of independent professionals and institutions with apparently infinite capacities for adaptation.

As a result of this experience, the recent past has seen a growing interest in indirect forms of regulation that make public use of private interest. A number of serious proposals have been advanced to apply this approach to the medical care sector. The Health Maintenance Organization movement of the early 1970s can be seen in this light. Enthoven's well-publicized consumer-choice proposal for national health insurance was also of this type (see Enthoven, 1978). The difficulty with both of these efforts has been the extent to which they have relied, first, on the creation of complex new organizations and, second, on fundamental changes by the public in choosing to give up attachments to their family doctors in favor of a "more rational," organized, and prepaid form of care.

The principal advantage of the proposal advanced here over these plans is that, while it retains the theoretical advantages of prepayment, it makes use of the existing private practice medical care system. It places the ordinary primary care physician at risk (instead of the HMO) for the patient's medical care and provides him or her with the same incentives that obtain in the organization model. But it permits citizens to remain with their family physicians. Moreover, if it works, it might lead to a more efficient system by promoting organized relationships among currently independent providers. And, finally, it might even help to solve the problem of maldistribution of physicians by encouraging young physicians to choose primary care over specialties and to locate in underserved areas.

The promise is great. The proposal has theoretical advantages and it appears to be practical. All that is needed is the leadership to give it a fair test.

Appendix A
New York State Medicaid Application and Instructions

REDI—REFERENCE GUIDE

Application/Recertification of Need for Medical Assistance

When you apply for Medical Assistance from the Department of Social Services because you do not have money to meet your medical needs, you must fill out a special form called Application for Medical Assistance. When you return to the Social Services Department to review this form with a worker, you must bring with you certain items to prove statements made in your application.

EVERY STATEMENT MADE IN YOUR APPLICATION MUST BE VERIFIED BY YOU BEFORE MEDICAID COVERAGE CAN BE APPROVED. The following list indicates what documents, statements, or papers must be brought at the time of interview:

SECTION A: **Verification of Residence (Where you live)**
Current utility bill (telephone, LILCO, oil etc.,) **OR** Mortgage statement **OR** statement from landlord verifying your address. Residence of children must also be verified; letter from school, physician's note or statement from responsible adult outside of immediate family must be used.

SECTION B: **Verification of Dates and Places of Birth of all Family Members**
Birth Certificates **OR** Baptismal Certificates **OR** Passports. Verification must show relationship of children to parent(s).

Verification of Social Security Number
Social Security card **OR** Railroad Retirment claim number.

Verification of Date of Last Move to New York State
Copy of lease agreement; receipt of deposit on utilities, for example.

Verification of Marital Status
Submit whatever applies: Marriage Certificate; Separation papers, Divorce decree; Death Certificate.

SECTION D: **Verification of Driver's License Number**
Driver's licenses for both husband and wife.

SECTION F: **Verification of Pregnancy**
Doctor's note confirming pregnancy and stating expected delivery date.

SECTION G: **Verification of Current Disability**
Our Agency may ask to have your family doctor complete our medical form stating diagnosis, etc. You will be advised at your interview for Medicaid if this information is needed.

SECTION J: **Verification of Veteran's Claim Number**
Document from Veteran's Administration stating VA Claim number and benefits available.

SECTION J1:   **Verification of Status of Foreign-Born Family Members**
Bring whatever applies: Naturalization papers; Alien registration card; passport; visa; name and address of sponsoring citizen (for aliens in residence less than 5 consecutive years).

SECTION K: **Verification of Housing Expenses**
Area 1 - Submit current rent receipt and any other bills incurred on rental **OR**
Area 2 - Verification of rent paid, or written statement from relative regarding applicant's contribution toward household expenses, **OR**
Area 3 - Mortgage statement and Tax Statement; Maintenance bills (last paid utility bills). We may need to see the deed to house.

SECTION L and M: **Verification of Earned Income**
Consecutive pay stubs for prior eight weeks, **OR** statement from employer listing gross income and all deductions for last eight weeks, **OR** if self-employed, you may submit current 3 month profit and loss statement or statements from all contractors you worked for during the last eight weeks.

SECTION O: **Verification of Union Membership**
Union book and statement from Union verifying all benefits available.

SECTION P: **Verification of Amounts of ALL Income received**
Submit whatever applies: Photocopy of Social Security check or statement from Social Security Administration's Office of amount received; Unemployment booklet; Workmen's Compensation award letter; Photocopy of any checks received, such as: Veteran's check, Union check, NYS Disability check, Pension check, Dividend check.

Court ordered or voluntary support statement from Family court or from separation or divorce papers. Documented amount of income from rental of rooms, an apartment, or a house, income from room and board, income from relatives or friends. Submit cancelled checks, etc. Verification of all other income. If you have applied for, but have not yet received certain benefits, bring proof of date of application.

SECTION Q and R: Verification of Status of Legally Responsible Relative

See Section B (Bring separation/divorce papers; if husband/wife is deceased, bring Death Certificate).

SECTION R: Verification of Details of Court Ordered Support Payments

Statement from Family Court giving Docket Number and amount of support.

SECTION T: Verification of Value of ALL Resources

Bring with you whatever applies: ALL bankbooks, including savings, checking, trust accounts, etc.; Credit Union statement; Stock and Bond Certificates and current market value per statement from stockbroker or attorney; Trust Fund account; Life Insurance policies and statement of current cash value of each, if not shown on policies.

SECTION U: Verification of Real Property

Deed to real estate, **OR** Assessment by real estate agent or appraisor stating current estimated market value.

SECTION V: Verification of Real/Personal Property transferred

Bring proof of transfer (bank accounts, stocks, bonds, legal papers describing transfer of all property.

SECTION X: Verification of Medicare Coverage

Medicare Card.

SECTION Y: Verification of any Health Insurance Coverage, including Coverage carried by Absent Parent of Spouse.

Health Insurance Identification Card **OR** Statement from insurance company giving policy number and which family members are covered.

PLEASE NOTE: BOTH HUSBAND AND WIFE ARE REQUIRED BY STATE LAW TO SIGN THE APPLICATION.

A SAMPLE OF THE NEW YORK
STATE MEDICAID APPLICATION
FOLLOWS ON PAGES 159–166

SOCIAL SERVICES DISTRICT AND/OR CENTER

FORM DSS-515 (REV. 1/77)

- FOR AGENCY USE ONLY -

| APPLICATION DATE Mo. | Day | Yr. | NEW ☐ REOPEN ☐ RECERT. ☐ | CROSS REFER/NO. | CASE NAME | CASE NUMBER - |

APPLICATION FOR MEDICAL ASSISTANCE

NEW YORK STATE DEPARTMENT OF SOCIAL SERVICES

Please Print clearly and complete all items. If answers are yes, give required details. If additional space is needed, see page 10.

At your interview you are required to supply proof of statements made in this application, including identity, age, place of residence, income and resources.

When Application is Completed and Signed, take or mail it to:

NOTE: ● The law provides for a fine or imprisonment, or both, for a person hiding facts or not telling the truth.

● A Face to Face interview is required.

(Name, Address and Telephone Number of the Social Services Department)

PART I. FAMILY AND RELATIVE DATA

| APPLICANT'S NAME (Last, First, M.I.) | MAIDEN NAME | OTHER NAMES BY WHICH KNOWN | VERIFICATION DATA (For Agency Use Only) DOCUMENTATION REQUIRED |
| ☐ MR. ☐ MRS. ☐ MISS | | | |

| APPLICANT LIVES AT (No., Street, Floor, Apt. No., City, County, Zip Code) | | TELEPHONE NUMBER | |

| MAILING ADDRESS OF APPLICANT (if same as above print same) (No., Street, Floor, Apt. No., City, County, Zip Code) | | IN CARE OF | |

| PERMANENT ADDRESS OF APPLICANT (if same as above print same) (No., Street, Floor, Apt. No., City, County, Zip Code) | | | |

TYPE OF ASSISTANCE	CASE NAME	CASE NUMBER	LAST DATE RECEIVED Mo. Day Yr.	AGENCY OR CENTER	
A	I ☐ Do ☐ Did ☐ Never Applied ☐ Received or For Public Assistance					
	I ☐ Do ☐ Did ☐ Never Applied ☐ Received or For Medicaid					
	I ☐ Do ☐ Did ☐ Never Applied ☐ Received or For Food Stamps					

I am applying for Medical Assistance because:

List any unpaid medical expenses for medical services provided within the past 3 calendar months:

Type of Service (Doctor, hospital, dental care, drugs, etc.)	Person Receiving Services	Date of Service

FORM DSS-515 (REV. 1/77)

Page 2

List in this section ALL persons usually living in your home, even if in a hospital or nursing home, or away at school.

FULL NAME (First, Middle, Last)	Social Security Number or Railroad Retirement Number (See Note Below)		Relation-ship To Me	SEX M/F	Birthdate Mo. Day Yr.	PLACE OF BIRTH (City and State)	MARITAL STATUS Married Single Widowed Separated Divorced	Date You Moved to NY State Mo. Day Yr.	Applying for Medical Assistance Yes No	DOCUMENTATION REQUIRED FOR APPLICANTS
		Suffix								
SELF										
HUSBAND/WIFE										

B

NOTE: If you are receiving Social Security benefits, enter the identification number printed on your monthly check or "Medicare" ID Card. If you are not receiving benefits, enter the number from your Social Security card.

If this application is for a person under age 21, complete the following:

MY FATHER'S NAME (Last, First) — ADDRESS

MY MOTHER'S NAME (Last, First) — ADDRESS

C

If person under 21 is married, complete the following:

MY HUSBAND/WIFE'S FATHER'S NAME (Last, First) — ADDRESS

MY HUSBAND/WIFE'S MOTHER'S NAME (Last, First) — ADDRESS

Do any of the applicants have a driver's license? ☐ Yes ☐ No

NAME — DRIVERS IDENTIFICATION NUMBER

D

Are any of the applicants or the husband or wife of any applicant in a hospital, nursing home, or other type of institution? ☐ Yes ☐ No

NAME OF PERSON — RELATIONSHIP — NAME AND ADDRESS OF INSTITUTION — DATE ADM.

E

Are any of the applicants pregnant? ☐ Yes ☐ No (Submit doctor's statement confirming delivery date)

NAME OF PREGNANT PERSON — MONTH BABY IS DUE

F

Page 3

FORM SSA-515 REV. 1/77

G Are any of the applicants blind, sick or disabled? ☐ Yes ☐ No

PERSON'S NAME	TYPE OF DISABILITY OR SICKNESS	DATE DISABILITY BEGAN	NAME AND ADDRESS OF DOCTOR OR CLINIC

H Are any of the applicants addicts or in a drug treatment program? ☐ Yes ☐ No

PERSON'S NAME	NAME AND ADDRESS OF DRUG PROGRAM BEING ATTENDED	ENTERED Mo. Yr.

I Has any applicant been in an institution, men.hosp., school for retarded and discharged/released on or after 6/29/74? ☐ Yes ☐ No

PERSON'S NAME	NAME, ADDRESS AND TYPE OF FACILITY	ENTERED Mo. Yr.	RELEASED Mo. Yr.

J Are any applicants veterans, or widow(er)s or children of a veteran? ☐ Yes ☐ No

FIRST NAME	NAME OF VETERAN (If a relative)	RELATIONSHIP	ARMED FORCES SERIAL NUMBER	VA CLAIM NUMBER

J-1 For any person listed in Section B who was not born in the U.S., complete the following:

FULL NAME (First, Middle Initial, Last)	NAME OF COUNTRY ENTERED FROM	PORT OF ENTRY	DATE ENTERED U.S.	If on Temp. Visa Date Until Admitted (Form 1-94)	STATUS (Check ✓ one and complete additional information requested)
HOUSEHOLD MEMBER					☐ Naturalized Citizen Certificate No. ____
MAIDEN NAME, if any					☐ Permanent Resident Alien - Alien Registration No. ____ Copy from Alien Card
SPONSORING CITIZEN (Name and Address)					☐ Temporary Non-Immigrant Alien Immigration File No., if any ____ ☐ Other, specify
HOUSEHOLD MEMBER					☐ Naturalized Citizen Certificate No. ____
MAIDEN NAME, if any					☐ Permanent Resident Alien - Alien Registration No. ____ Copy from Alien Card
SPONSORING CITIZEN (Name and Address)					☐ Temporary Non-Immigrant Alien Immigration File No., if any ____ ☐ Other, specify
HOUSEHOLD MEMBER					☐ Naturalized Citizen Certificate No. ____
MAIDEN NAME, if any					☐ Permanent Resident Alien - Alien Registration No. ____ Copy from Alien Card
SPONSORING CITIZEN (Name and Address)					☐ Temporary Non-Immigrant Alien Immigration File No., if any ____ ☐ Other, specify

FORM DSS-515 (REV. 1/77)   Page 4

PART II. LIVING ARRANGEMENTS

Area 1. If you pay rent, give the following:

NAME OF LANDLORD	HOW MANY PERSONS LIVE IN HOUSEHOLD	AMOUNT OF RENT	RENT RECEIPT FURNISHED
			☐ Yes ☐ No
ADDRESS OF LANDLORD		HEAT INCLUDED ☐ Yes ☐ No	TYPE OF FUEL USED	FUEL COST

DOCUMENTATION REQUIRED

Area 2. If you share a housing arrangement, or if you live in someone else's home, give the following information:

NAMES OF PERSONS YOU SHARE WITH	YOUR SHARE OF COST Amt. ____ per ____	NO. OF PERSONS LIVING IN YOUR HOME

RELATIONSHIP	ARE ANY OF THESE PERSONS ON PUBLIC ASSISTANCE? ☐ Yes ☐ No
	1. CASE NUMBER _____ AGENCY/CENTER _____
	2. CASE NUMBER _____ AGENCY/CENTER _____

IS THIS LIVING ARRANGEMENT	HEAT INCLUDED	TYPE OF FUEL USED	FUEL COST
☐ Permanent Mo. ___ Day ___ Yr.	☐ Yes ☐ No		
☐ Temporary – Date You Must Leave By:			

Area 3. If you own your own home check (✓) the one you have:

☐ House   ☐ Trailer/Mobile Home   ☐ Cooperative   ☐ Other (specify) _____

PURCHASE PRICE	DATE OF PURCHASE	ASSESSED VALUATION (from the bill)

NAME OF PERSON PAYING MORTGAGE	MORTGAGE PAID TO: (Name and Address)

MONTHLY MORTGAGE PAYMENT	DATE MORTGAGE LAST PAID Mo. ___ Day ___ Yr.	PROPERTY TAX Amount ____ Per ____	SCHOOL TAX Amount ____ Per ____
Principal _____			
Interest _____			

FIRE INSURANCE	WATER	SEWER	OTHER MAINTENANCE EXPENSES (specify)
Amount _____	Amount _____	Amount _____	1. _____ Amount _____ per ____
Per _____	Per _____	Per _____	2. _____ Amount _____ per ____

ANNUAL HEATING COST	DO YOU RENT PART OF YOUR HOME? ☐ Yes ☐ No To Whom _____	NO. OF ROOMS	NO. OF ROOMS IN YOUR APARTMENT

SIZE OF LOT AND/OR ADJACENT LAND OWNED	HEAT INCLUDED ☐ Yes ☐ No	TYPE OF FUEL USED	FUEL COST

FORM DSS-515 (REV. 1/77)

Page 5

PART III. EMPLOYMENT

Are any of the applicants employed or self-employed (include all full-time, part-time, overtime and second jobs)
☐ Yes ☐ No   Show pay stubs for last eight weeks.

Name of Person	Name and Address of Employer	Date Started	Occupation	Gross Salary	Period (wk., etc.)	Amt. of Tips	DOCUMENTATION REQUIRED
L,							

List the following items which are withheld from wages. Enter amounts from latest pay stub.

FIRST NAME	INCOME TAX PAID OR WITHHELD			Social Security Tax (FICA)	HEALTH INS. PAID	Court Ordered Payments	DOCUMENTATION REQUIRED
	FEDERAL Amount	STATE Amount	CITY Amount	Amount	Amount	Amount	
M							

Was any applicant employed during the past 6 months (other than present employment)? ☐ Yes ☐ No

PERSON'S NAME	EMPLOYER'S NAME AND ADDRESS	PERIOD OF EMP. FROM Mo. Yr.	TO Mo. Yr.	GROSS SALARY Amount	Per	REASON FOR LEAVING
N						

Are any of the applicants a present or past union member? ☐ Yes ☐ No

PERSON'S NAME	NAME, ADDRESS AND PHONE NO. OF UNION	DATE JOINED Mo. Yr.	DATE LEFT Mo. Yr.
O			

FORM DSS-515 (REV. 1/77)

Page 6

PART IV. OTHER INCOME

Do any of the applicants have or expect to receive any of the following? ☐ Yes ☐ No

TYPE OF BENEFIT	Applied Yes No	Date Applied Mo. Day Yr.	Receiving Yes No	NAME OF PERSON RECEIVING INCOME	AMOUNT	WEEKLY MONTHLY YEARLY	DOCUMENTATION REQUIRED
Unemployment Insurance							
Workmen's Compensation							
Veteran's Benefits or Pension							
Social Security							
Union Benefits							
Railroad Retirement							
NYS Disability Insurance							
Court Order/Support Payments							
Income From: Rent, Produce of Farm, Roomers, Boarders, Mortgages, etc.							
GI Dependency Allotment							
Income from Relative or Friend (Give name)							
Employer Pensions							
Dividends from stocks, bonds or Life Insurance and interest from bank accounts							
G.I. Bill							
Income from Training Program							
Other Income							

Do any of the applicants have a legal husband/wife living elsewhere? ☐ Yes ☐ No

NAME OF MARRIED PERSON IN HOUSEHOLD AND NAME OF LEGAL HUSBAND/WIFE	ADDRESS OF LEGAL HUSBAND/WIFE	SO. SEC. NO. OF HUSBAND/WIFE	SUP-PORT PAID	If Yes, Amount/per	If No, Are You Willing To Seek Support
MARRIED PERSON			☐ Yes ☐ No		☐ Yes ☐ No
LEGAL HUSBAND/WIFE					
NAME AND ADDRESS OF PRESENT OR LAST KNOWN EMPLOYER OF HUSBAND/WIFE					

Page 7

Are there any parents of children living outside the home?   (Include the father of unborn child)   ☐ Yes   ☐ No

R

1

ABSENT PARENT'S NAME	SOCIAL SECURITY NO.	HOME ADDRESS		

PLACE OF EMPLOYMENT		AUTOMOBILE LICENSE NUMBER	

FIRST NAME OF EACH CHILD THAT BELONGS TO THE ABSENT PARENT
1.   2.   3.   4.   5.

SUPPORT PAID	SUPPORT	LOCATION OF COURT	DOCKET NO.
Amount _____	☐ Voluntary		
Per _____	☐ Court Order		

DATE PARENT LEFT HOME   Mo. ___ Yr. ___

Is this absent parent receiving public assistance?   ☐ Yes   ☐ No

AGENCY/CENTER	CASE NUMBER	WILL YOU SEEK SUPPORT ☐ Yes ☐ No

2

ABSENT PARENT'S NAME	SOCIAL SECURITY NO.	HOME ADDRESS		

PLACE OF EMPLOYMENT		AUTOMOBILE LICENSE NUMBER	

FIRST NAME OF EACH CHILD THAT BELONGS TO ABSENT PARENT
1.   2.   3.   4.   5.

SUPPORT PAID	SUPPORT	LOCATION OF COURT	DOCKET NO.
Amount _____	☐ Voluntary		
Per _____	☐ Court Order		

DATE PARENT LEFT HOME   Mo. ___ Yr. ___

Is this absent parent receiving public assistance?   ☐ Yes   ☐ No

AGENCY/CENTER	CASE NUMBER	WILL YOU SEEK SUPPORT ☐ Yes ☐ No

S

The following people live with me and are NOT applying for assistance:

FULL NAME (First, Middle Initial, Last)	RELATIONSHIP TO ME	Sex M/F	SELF-SUP-PORTING	If self-supporting, is he contributing to support of household	If Yes, Amount/per	If Already Receiving Public Assistance give	
						CASE NO.	CENTER/AGENCY
			☐ Yes ☐ No	☐ Yes ☐ No			
			☐ Yes ☐ No	☐ Yes ☐ No			
			☐ Yes ☐ No	☐ Yes ☐ No			
			☐ Yes ☐ No	☐ Yes ☐ No			

FORM DSS-515 (REV. 1/77)

Page 8

PART V. RESOURCES

Do any of the applicants have the following:

TYPE OF RESOURCE	Yes	No	NAME OF PERSON OWNING RESOURCE			VALUE OF RESOURCE	DOCUMENTATION REQUIRED
Cash on Hand							
Bank Account(s) 1			NAME AND ADDRESS OF BANK		ACCOUNT NO.		
2							
Pending Lawsuit Which May Result in Cash Award			NAME AND ADDRESS OF LAWYER				
Credit Union							
Stocks/Bonds							
Trust Fund							
Safe Deposit Box							
Union Benefits (Including Life or Health Insurance)							
Other (Specify)							

T

Life Insurance 1	INSURED	INSURANCE CO.	POLICY NO.	FACE VALUE	CASH VALUE
	TYPE OF INSURANCE	BENEFICIARY	DATE OF ISSUE	PREMIUM	PERIOD
2	INSURED	INSURANCE CO.	POLICY NO.	FACE VALUE	CASH VALUE
	TYPE OF INSURANCE	BENEFICIARY	DATE OF ISSUE	PREMIUM	PERIOD
3	INSURED	INSURANCE CO.	POLICY NO.	FACE VALUE	CASH VALUE
	TYPE OF INSURANCE	BENEFICIARY	DATE OF ISSUE	PREMIUM	PERIOD
Burial Fund	NAME OF PERSON OWNING RESOURCE			VALUE OF RESOURCE	

Do any of the applicants own property other than listed in Section K?   ☐ Yes   ☐ No

DESCRIPTION OF PROPERTY	VALUE OF PROPERTY

U

LOCATION OF PROPERTY

Appendix B
Tables A1 through A18

Table A-1. State Expenditures for Selected Purposes, 1965–1976

	1965	1966	1967	1968	1969	1970	1971	1972	1973	1974	1975	1976
All Purposes	45,507	51,043	58,610	66,254	74,218	85,055	98,840	109,243	118,836	132,134	156,171	181,966
Education	14,532	17,749	21,229	24,279	27,162	30,865	35,092	38,348	41,599	46,860	54,012	59,630
Public welfare	5,434	6,020	7,188	8,649	10,866	13,206	16,278	19,191	21,678	22,538	22,559	29,633
Highways	9,844	10,349	11,284	11,848	12,518	13,483	14,810	15,380	15,025	15,847	17,483	18,100

Percent Increase

	1965–66	1966–67	1967–68	1968–69	1969–70	1970–71	1971–72	1972–73	1973–74	1974–75	1975–76	1965–76
All purposes	12.2	14.8	13.0	12.0	14.6	16.2	10.5	8.8	11.2	18.2	16.5	299.9
Education	22.1	19.6	14.4	11.9	13.6	13.7	9.3	8.5	12.6	15.3	10.4	310.3
Public welfare	10.8	19.4	20.3	25.6	21.5	23.3	17.9	13.0	4.0	—	31.4	445.3
Highways	5.1	9.0	5.0	5.8	7.7	9.8	3.8	-2.3	5.5	10.3	3.5	83.9

Expenditures for Selected Purposes as Percent of All State Expenditures

	1965	1966	1967	1968	1969	1970	1971	1972	1973	1974	1975	1976
All purposes	100.0	100.0	100.0	100.0	100.0	100.0	100.0	100.0	100.0	100.0	100.0	100.0
Education	31.9	34.8	36.2	36.6	36.6	36.3	35.5	35.1	35.0	35.5	34.6	32.8
Public welfare	11.9	11.8	12.3	13.1	14.6	15.5	16.5	17.6	18.2	17.1	14.5	16.3
Highways	21.6	20.3	19.3	17.9	16.9	15.9	15.0	14.1	12.6	12.0	11.2	9.9

Source: Bureau of the Census, State Government Finances, Annual Reports, 1965–1976, U.S. Department of Commerce; table 9.

Table A-2.   State Intergovernmental Revenues, Selected Purposes, 1965–1976

	1965	1966	1967	1968	1969	1970	1971	1972	1973	1974	1975	1976
From Federal Government (in millions of dollars)												
Total	9,874	11,743	13,616	15,228	16,907	19,252	22,754	26,791	31,353	31,632	36,148	42,013
Education	1,393	2,654	3,500	3,891	4,121	4,554	5,468	5,984	6,430	6,720	7,879	8,661
Public welfare	3,133	3,573	4,353	5,240	6,477	7,818	9,553	12,289	13,653	13,320	14,248	16,867
Highways	3,987	3,972	4,033	4,198	4,201	4,431	4,814	4,871	4,648	4,503	5,260	6,262

Percent Increase	1965-66	1966-67	1967-68	1968-69	1969-70	1970-71	1971-72	1972-73	1973-74	1974-75	1975-76
Total	18.9	15.9	11.8	11.0	13.9	18.2	17.7	17.0	<0.01	14.3	16.2
Education	90.5	31.9	11.2	5.9	10.5	20.1	9.4	7.5	4.5	17.2	9.9
Public welfare	14.0	21.8	20.4	23.6	20.7	22.2	28.6	11.1	-2.4	7.0	18.4
Highways	-<0.01	1.5	4.1	<0.01	5.5	8.6	1.2	-4.6	-3.1	16.8	19.1

	1965	1966	1967	1968	1969	1970	1971	1972	1973	1974	1975	1976
From Local Governments (in millions of dollars)												
Total	447	503	673	707	868	995	1,054	1,191	1,339	1,538	1,680	2,704
Education	52	59	64	74	85	90	107	116	136	144	182	223
Public Welfare	34	39	77	79	233	278	290	322	357	482	532	606
Highways	145	155	243	192	174	165	158	185	186	207	245	248

Percent Increase	1965-66	1966-67	1967-68	1968-69	1969-70	1970-71	1971-72	1972-73	1973-74	1974-75	1975-76
Total	12.5	33.8	5.1	22.8	14.6	5.9	13.0	12.4	14.9	9.2	61.0
Education	13.5	8.5	15.6	14.9	5.9	18.9	8.4	17.2	5.9	26.4	22.5
Public welfare	14.7	97.4	2.6	194.9	19.3	4.3	11.0	10.9	35.0	10.4	13.9
Highways	6.9	56.8	-21.0	-9.4	-5.2	-4.2	17.1	<0.01	11.3	18.4	1.2

Table A-2. Continued

Totals (in millions of dollars)

	1965	1966	1967	1968	1969	1970	1971	1972	1973	1974	1975	1976
Total	21	12,246	14,289	15,935	17,775	20,247	23,808	27,982	32,692	33,170	37,828	44,717
Education	1,445	2,713	3,564	3,965	4,206	4,644	5,575	6,100	6,566	6,864	8,061	8,884
Public welfare	3,167	3,612	4,430	5,319	6,710	8,096	9,843	12,611	14,010	13,802	14,780	17,473
Highways	4,132	4,127	4,276	4,390	4,375	4,596	4,972	5,056	4,834	4,710	5,505	6,510

Percent Increase

	1965–66	1966–67	1967–68	1968–69	1969–70	1970–71	1971–72	1972–73	1973–74	1974–75	1975–76
Total	18.7	16.7	11.5	11.5	13.9	17.6	17.5	16.8	1.5	14.0	18.2
Education	87.8	31.4	11.3	6.1	10.4	20.0	9.4	7.6	4.5	17.4	10.2
Public welfare	14.1	22.6	20.1	26.2	20.7	21.6	28.1	11.1	-1.5	7.1	18.2
Highways	$-<0.01$	3.6	2.7	$-<0.01$	5.1	8.2	1.7	-4.4	-2.6	16.9	18.3

Source: Bureau of Census, State Government Finances, Annual Reports, 1965–1976, U.S. Department of Commerce, table 7.

Table A-3. State Revenues for Selected Purposes, 1965–1976[a]

(in millions of dollars)

	1965	1966	1967	1968	1969	1970	1971	1972	1973	1974	1975	1976
Total	35,186	38,797	44,321	50,319	56,443	64,808	75,032	81,261	86,144	98,964	118,343	137,249
Education	13,087	15,036	17,665	20,314	22,956	26,221	29,517	32,248	35,033	39,996	45,951	50,746
Public welfare	2,267	2,408	2,758	3,330	4,156	5,110	6,435	6,580	7,668	8,736	7,779	12,160
Highways	5,712	6,222	7,008	7,458	8,143	8,887	9,838	10,324	10,191	11,137	11,978	11,590

Percent Increase

	1965-66	1966-67	1967-68	1968-69	1969-70	1970-71	1971-72	1972-73	1973-74	1974-75	1975-76	1965-76
Total	10.3	14.2	13.5	12.2	14.8	15.8	8.3	6.0	14.9	19.6	16.0	290.1
Education	14.9	17.5	15.0	13.0	14.2	12.6	9.3	8.6	14.2	14.9	10.4	287.8
Public welfare	6.2	14.5	20.7	24.8	23.0	25.9	2.3	16.5	13.9	-11.0	56.3	436.4
Highways	8.9	12.6	6.4	9.2	9.1	10.7	4.9	-1.3	9.3	7.6	-3.2	102.9

Dollar Increase

	1965-66	1966-67	1967-68	1968-69	1969-70	1970-71	1971-72	1972-73	1973-74	1974-75	1975-76	1965-76
Total	3,611	5,524	5,998	6,124	8,365	10,224	6,229	4,883	12,820	19,379	18,906	102,063
Education	1,949	2,629	2,649	2,642	3,265	3,296	2,731	2,785	4,963	5,955	4,795	37,659
Public welfare	141	350	572	826	954	1,325	145	1,088	1,068	-957	4,381[b]	9,893
Highways	510	786	450	685	744	951	486	-133	946	841	-388	5,878

[a]Calculated by subtracting Intergovernmental Revenues by Function (Table A–2) from Total State Expenditures by Function.(Table A–1.)

[b]1974–1976 increase in state revenues for public welfare was $3,424,000,000, an annual increase of $1,712,000,000.

Table A–4.   Increase in State Revenues for Selected Purposes (in millions) 1965–1976

	In Dollars	In Percent
Total	102,063	100.0
Education	37,659	36.9
Public welfare	9,893	9.7
Highways	5,878	5.8
Other	48,633	47.6

Table A–5.   Utilization of Hospital Services, 1972–1976

	1972	1973	1974
Recipients Discharged			
Aged	352,281	18,976[a]	139,269[b]
Blind			
Disabled	1,339,022	312,390	329,115
AFDC adults		695,011	709,127
AFDC children	789,918	705,326	741,185
All	2,511,472	1,764,579	1,751,579
Total Discharges			
Aged	500,926	28,942[a]	181,463[b]
Blind			
Disabled	1,919,415	469,873	508,088
AFDC adults		893,893	919,276
AFDC children	988,260	826,887	898,344
All	3,448,772	2,287,903	2,305,271
Days of Care			
Aged	6,271,067	243,699[a]	1,957,136[b]
Blind			
Disabled	17,948,004	5,093,066	5,961,768
AFDC adults		5,316,730	5,493,275
AFDC children	5,723,517	4,413,331	4,882,206
All	30,244,015	16,956,283	18,415,611
Discharges per 1,000 Recipients			
Aged	1,422	1,525	1,303
Blind			
Disabled	1,433	1,504	1,544
AFDC adults		1,286	1,296
AFDC children	1,251	1,172	1,212
All	1,373	1,296	1,316
Days of Care per Discharge			
Aged	12.5	8.4	10.8
Blind			
Disabled	9.4	10.8	11.7
AFDC Adults		5.9	6.0
AFDC children	5.8	5.3	5.4
All	8.8	7.4	8.0

Source: NCSS (later, HCFA), Report B-4 and B-4 Supplement, 1972–1976. While these data are less complete than those reported in Tables 3–1 and 3–2, they reflect reports from more than forty states in each instance, except for the two noted. It would be misleading to compare any data but rates per recipient or per discharge, however, because the nonreporting states varied from year to year.
[a]1973 Aged, 19 states.
[b]1974 Aged, 29 states.
[c]Percent change, 1973–1976.

Table A–5. Continued

1975	1976	Percent Change 1972–1976
321,645	268,647	
334,104	394,301	
732,398	783,948	
717,825	792,481	
2,335,959	2,452,395	
406,414	357,507	
506,902	632,735	
975,799	1,026,920	
868,670	969,895	
3,030,557	3,261,359	
5,247,911	3,480,266	
5,340,893	6,334,645	
5,610,031	5,580,441	
4,612,471	4,802,796	
22,940,572	22,673,725	
1,264	1,331	−6.4
1,517	1,605	+6.7[c]
1,332	1,310	+1.9[c]
1,210	1,224	−2.2
1,297	1,330	−3.1
12.9	9.7	−22.4
10.5	10.0	−7.4[c]
5.7	5.4	−8.5[c]
5.3	5.0	−13.8
7.6	7.0	−20.5

Table A-6   Utilization of Physician Services

	1972	1973	1974	1975	1976	Percent Change 1972–1976
Recipients Using Physician Services						
Aged	2,008,599	1,802,712	2,007,438	1,984,904	2,028,146	
Blind	64,345	58,402	75,252	59,510	55,954	
Disabled	983,362	918,361	1,244,689	1,250,948	1,430,470	
AFDC adults	2,196,041	2,371,036	2,732,919	2,853,534	2,872,241	
AFDC children	5,471,958	5,130,223	5,636,699	5,616,466	5,742,235	
All	11,854,382	11,309,407	12,745,582	13,077,387	13,600,492	
Total Physician Visits						
Aged	16,598,888	14,349,492	13,756,786	13,198,909	13,401,757	
Blind	465,858	473,760	492,830	409,372	371,292	
Disabled	9,270,176	9,054,451	10,436,173	10,690,793	12,684,580	
AFDC adults	13,686,799	15,056,025	17,323,362	19,506,345	19,499,377	
AFDC children	20,660,282	20,341,203	22,120,738	23,453,976	25,037,679	
All	65,507,769	63,081,488	68,715,438	73,558,512	77,715,359	
Average Physician Visits per Recipient						
Aged	8.3	8.0	6.9	6.7	6.6	−20.5
Blind	7.2	8.1	6.6	6.9	6.6	−8.3
Disabled	9.4	9.9	8.4	8.6	8.9	−5.3
AFDC adults	6.2	6.3	6.3	6.8	6.8	9.7
AFDC children	3.8	4.0	3.9	4.2	4.4	15.8
All	5.5	5.6	5.4	5.6	5.7	7.3

Table A-7. Utilization of Extended Care Facilities

	1972	1973	1974	1975	1976	Percent Change 1972–1976	Percent Change 1973–1976
A. Skilled Nursing Facilities							
Recipients Discharged							
Aged	417,622	410,153	362,747	334,448	365,100		
Disabled	89,706	90,154	78,868	65,839	73,221		
All	543,407	520,096	453,609	408,674	455,102		
Total Days of Care							
Aged	81,180,782	75,855,519	68,597,833	65,017,971	69,029,461		
Disabled	17,442,750	15,528,802	14,528,104	11,782,169	13,031,274		
All	105,945,600	94,429,397	84,964,323	78,110,582	84,447,587		
Days of Care per Recipient							
Aged	194.4	184.9	189.1	194.4	189.1	−2.7	2.3
Disabled	194.4	172.2	184.2	179.0	178.0	−8.4	3.4
All	195.0	181.6	187.3	191.1	185.6	−4.8	2.2
B. Intermediate Care Facilities							
Recipients Discharged							
Aged		246,688	332,966	382,175	438,798		
Disabled		—	—	—	—		
All		335,782	465,300	503,583	580,121		
Total Days of Care							
Aged		51,684,270	77,280,258	95,184,545	108,459,189		
Disabled		—	—	—	—		
All		70,932,213	108,211,083	121,604,397	142,399,300		
Days of Care per Recipient							
Aged		209.5	232.1	249.1	247.2	18.0	
Disabled		—	—	—	—	—	
All		211.2	232.6	241.5	245.5	16.2	

Table A–8. Utilization of Prescription Drugs

	1972	1973	1974	1975	1976	Percent Change 1972–1976
Recipients						
Aged	2,201,620	1,946,612	2,325,545	2,164,800	2,400,639	26.6
Blind	68,017	61,630	86,462	61,357	59,869	26.1
Disabled	1,046,564	931,877	1,338,216	1,254,907	1,510,684	25.1
AFDC adults	2,114,778	2,311,163	2,647,758	2,611,269	2,790,584	13.9
AFDC children	4,435,524	4,072,778	4,720,672	4,519,838	4,947,665	25.0
All	10,884,076	10,014,172	14,307,772	11,658,286	12,809,786	30.4
Prescriptions						
Aged	40,577,219	42,230,485	45,690,441	51,775,439	56,042,932	
Blind	1,038,362	1,176,324	1,839,617	1,163,299	1,157,871	
Disabled	18,297,226	19,543,059	23,988,423	27,041,520	33,100,473	
AFDC adults	16,708,862	21,868,411	24,115,839	25,116,286	25,144,724	
AFDC children	17,536,129	17,055,177	20,448,220	19,853,747	24,569,533	
All	100,314,573	106,165,519	120,830,811	130,971,754	151,459,593	
Average Prescriptions per Recipient						
Aged	18.4	21.7	19.7	23.9	23.3	
Blind	15.3	19.1	21.3	19.0	19.3	
Disabled	17.5	21.0	17.9	21.6	21.9	
AFDC adults	7.9	9.5	9.1	9.6	9.0	
AFDC children	4.0	4.2	4.3	4.4	5.0	
All	9.2	10.6	8.5	11.2	11.8	

Table A-9. Medicaid Eligibles, Recipients, and Expenditures for Grant Recipients Only, Selected Categories, Selected States, Selected Years (in thousands)

	CY 1968			CY 1970			FY 1972			FY 1974			FY 1976		
	Eligibles	Recipients	Expenditures	Eligibles	Recipients	Expenditures	Eligibles	Recipients	Expenditures	Eligibles	Recipients	Expenditures	Eligibles	Recipients	Expenditures
A. Elderly															
Indiana	17.9	20.9	17,859	16.3	18.3	5,574.2	16.0	18.6	5,456.9	18.7	15.3	15,011.0	21.7	12.5	18,504.2
Iowa	23.8	26.5	6,642	23.9	27.4	6,130.3	21.7	25.0	5,190.1	14.4	15.1	8,831.2	16.0	16.8	12,161.5
Nebraska	8.4	9.1	4,169	8.0	8.9	2,066.4	7.3	7.5	2,328.0	7.5	4.6	2,564.3	8.3	6.9	7,106.0
Texas	229.5	179.0	62,170	232.5	193.4	50,966.7	218.4	208.4	58,206.3	181.1	177.6	102,411.7	186.4	199.8	143,350.6
California	292.5	374.0	124,712	316.5	801.2	187,128.7	309.6	738.3	107,322.0	295.0	731.5	145,532.9	330.7	514.6	225,568.4
Massachusetts	48.6	66.8	24,008	51.7	n.a.	n.a.	57.6	n.a.	n.a.	65.5	115.9	47,419.5	79.0	76.1	45,424.7
New York	76.4	112.0	199,414	96.6	216.1	245,345.1	113.9	215.5	142,879.0	132.2	216.4	154,321.5	170.2	291.2	202,213.4
Georgia	90.0	70.7	18,134	92.3	94.6	25,653.8	91.3	92.0	22,582.3	89.9	85.5	29,750.6	91.1	117.4	44,679.7
Oklahoma	78.6	68.7	29,069	73.8	65.2	35,517.6	66.6	64.8	38,366.9	52.8	65.1	32,509.5	49.6	49.2	57,046.1
Tennessee	50.6	55.7	11,797	53.1	48.8	7,879.1	49.1	47.7	8,419.4	63.3	50.8	17,747.4	77.7	77.5	31,885.7
Colorado	39.5	n.a.	n.a.	35.8	59.6	19,526.0	31.1	29.6	7,861.9	22.2	22.2	29,898.5	19.3	28.7	36,916.1
Maryland	7.8	8.4	2,873	8.5	11.7	4,267.1	9.8	13.8	5,550.0	14.6	11.0	8,194.8	18.8	15.7	11,748.9
Pennsylvania	43.6	n.a.	n.a.	48.6	58.4	13,743.5	50.4	50.1	17,013.5	52.5	66.9	59,408.2	64.6	65.8	56,937.1
B. Disabled															
Indiana	3.1	4.4	5,635	5.2	6.5	5,244.6	9.1	10.5	10,778.2	13.7	12.7	21,570.4	20.9	10.9	22,015.6
Iowa	2.3	3.0	2,421	3.1	3.8	1,874.6	3.5	4.0	1,887.8	5.3	4.0	4,645.5	12.2	12.2	17,887.1
Nebraska	3.4	3.6	3,888	4.4	5.3	3,781.3	5.8	6.1	5,066.1	6.3	5.6	6,323.4	7.4	6.3	11,673.7
Texas	14.9	11.0	8,038	23.3	17.8	20,461.3	25.9	28.5	23,787.0	41.4	34.6	35,749.5	89.0	87.6	121,332.1
California	123.5	181.0	137,514	172.0	458.4	248,944.3	197.6	463.3	225,705.7	235.6	594.4	334,794.2	327.0	480.6	481,681.1
Massachusetts	14.8	22.0	17,231	16.7	n.a.	n.a.	22.0	n.a.	n.a.	33.4	71.2	57,619.7	48.2	48.5	75,481.1
New York	56.7	57.0	79,247	78.2	129.3	135,369.9	152.7	162.6	240,069.0	178.7	229.2	285,744.0	220.4	260.2	377,540.9
Georgia	29.4	25.1	9,841	33.3	38.3	25,130.4	40.7	42.7	-32,630.7	45.8	42.3	37,500.5	70.6	79.1	65,640.5
Oklahoma	19.7	16.3	11,237	21.4	19.2	14,643.2	24.1	21.7	17,748.5	24.8	22.6	18,542.8	32.3	21.4	28,839.5
Tennessee	18.4	2.9	1,116	24.5	22.2	6,435.7	28.4	25.5	10,042.6	37.5	30.0	18,769.1	58.6	54.8	43,229.2
Colorado	7.2	n.a.	n.a.	9.3	17.6	9,701.2	12.9	14.1	9,963.3	13.6	18.7	25,315.2	15.2	14.3	28,725.8
Maryland	13.1	14.2	6,618	16.1	19.7	10,734.8	18.6	21.3	16,014.6	26.8	27.1	28,161.6	29.1	27.2	29,970.1
Pennsylvania	26.0	n.a.	n.a.	37.1	43.3	24,806.6	33.3	54.2	31,638.4	51.9	88.3	53,773.4	82.0	185.6	85,301.1

C. AFDC children

Indiana	40.0	33.0	1,828	63.2	54.4	4,801.9	122.5	111.3	16,672.8	119.9	121.2	17,403.0	129.3	130.0	26,263.5
Iowa	37.5	39.7	4,158	49.0	53.7	5,529.5	59.2	66.8	8,936.9	56.4	68.9	9,801.2	65.7	63.3	14,111.7
Nebraska	18.7	15.1	744	24.5	22.1	2,722.8	30.7	29.0	4,130.1	28.1	27.2	4,279.4	25.6	27.9	5,140.9
Texas	104.5	54.4	4,306	193.0	79.1	16,737.3	323.0	222.7	30,126.1	309.4	277.4	41,098.9	251.6	257.9	50,720.7
California	592.5	841.0	83,480	904.5	1,261.0	154,037.1	1,050.0	1,377.4	199,837.0	922.0	1,175.9	204,698.1	985.2	1,245.9	294,656.8
Massachusetts	110.5	99.6	10,181	166.5	n.a.	n.a.	202.2	n.a.	n.a.	212.6	335.6	52,200.1	250.7	314.2	96,158.1
New York	626.0	602.0	68,346	793.0	1,070.7	117,316.7	912.8	1,122.7	153,344.2	837.5	1,121.5	289,202.3	856.3	1,174.3	394,628.9
Georgia	87.7	39.1	2,438	167.0	116.8	10,120.8	238.1	160.4	15,321.2	255.0	196.5	25,251.2	210.4	238.8	31,532.3
Oklahoma	67.8	45.7	3,663	72.4	61.4	5,137.1	81.7	72.3	8,017.1	71.5	74.0	7,909.3	66.9	73.7	11,933.3
Tennessee	77.0	2.3	566	111.0	60.2	3,929.8	141.8	91.2	8,450.4	143.1	119.5	12,654.4	151.8	146.3	22,963.3
Colorado	42.3	n.a.	n.a.	55.3	46.7	4,152.5	74.3	44.5	5,427.7	68.5	44.8	8,025.0	67.5	61.6	11,309.2
Maryland	85.9	70.3	6,167	108.0	98.5	11,052.7	148.5	126.6	18,461.1	158.7	156.4	27,380.5	153.7	157.5	35,811.4
Pennsylvania	229.5	n.a.	n.a.	339.0	395.6	28,598.8	457.7	403.0	37,566.9	422.1	501.3	43,865.7	438.6	892.7	77,567.4

D. AFDC adults

Indiana	13.0	14.4	2,594	21.9	26.0	7,694.9	43.9	45.1	16,647.3	42.8	54.1	21,405.1	48.2	61.4	32,155.4
Iowa	13.9	13.8	4,106	19.2	24.7	7,492.2	24.6	23.9	7,969.3	24.5	25.9	9,283.2	30.8	38.0	18,864.2
Nebraska	5.7	5.8	857	8.0	9.6	2,999.6	10.9	12.6	4,526.8	10.1	11.4	4,592.2	10.2	12.3	5,818.3
Texas	32.0	29.3	7,270	63.5	42.6	22,368.8	114.0	124.0	46,126.9	109.8	126.1	53,165.0	86.9	100.6	56,383.3
California	224.0	401.0	101,764	379.5	714.1	198,348.5	458.8	587.2	164,976.4	404.4	621.6	225,657.5	450.5	604.3	289,331.4
Massachusetts	37.5	54.9	16,296	62.0	78.4	n.a.	78.4	n.a.	n.a.	92.6	152.7	59,457.9	111.7	149.0	44,934.4
New York	226.5	403.0	151,614	312.5	554.8	162,732.7	377.6	174.9	44,407.1	338.0	582.4	260,832.5	372.8	669.8	344,953.5
Georgia	26.4	21.9	3,906	54.0	57.5	16,229.6	83.4	81.5	25,469.2	91.1	99.6	36,342.0	72.5	106.8	35,180.0
Oklahoma	22.4	24.1	3,091	24.4	28.5	3,877.7	28.1	31.1	21,778.2	22.4	21.8	5,619.8	21.8	21.9	8,439.3
Tennessee	23.1	1.5	582	33.5	26.9	4,411.1	46.1	37.6	9,043.6	48.2	41.3	10,893.6	55.1	52.1	18,990.0
Colorado	13.3	n.a.	n.a.	19.7	28.8	5,746.0	29.3	27.1	6,256.1	26.5	22.8	8,829.9	28.7	24.1	12,443.6
Maryland	25.6	27.9	6,005	34.0	39.6	11,248.7	52.3	75.6	20,936.6	58.8	69.0	30,369.2	62.5	73.7	38,430.0
Pennsylvania	83.0	n.a.	n.a.	136.0	218.5	39,104.4	203.5	320.8	54,096.4	192.1	388.1	68,623.7	203.3	583.1	106,538.3

Table A-10.   Change in Eligibles, Recipients, and Expenditures (Per Capita) 1968-1976[a]

Pearson Correlations

	Elderly	Disabled	AFDC Adults	AFDC Children
Eligibles/Recipients				
Correlation coefficient	.638	.971	.863	.842
N	11	11	11	11
Significance	.017	.001	.001	.001
Eligibles/Expenditures				
Correlation coefficient	-.734	.897	.588	.585
N	11	11	11	11
Significance	.005	.001	.029	.029
Recipients/Expenditures				
Correlation coefficient	-.406	.877	.552	.709
N	11	11	11	11
Significance	.108	.001	.039	.007

[a]Colorado and Pennsylvania were omitted because of missing 1968 data.

Table A–11.   Change in Eligibles, Recipients, and Expenditures, Twelve States, 1970–1976[a]

Pearson Correlations

	Elderly	Disabled	AFDC Adults	AFDC Children
Eligibles/Recipients				
Correlation coefficient	.593	.547	.904	.620
N	12	12	12	12
Significance	.021	.033	.001	.016
Eligibles/Expenditures				
Correlation coefficient	−.648	.812	.440	.308
N	12	12	12	12
Significance	0.011	.001	.076	.165
Recipients/Expenditures				
Correlation coefficient	−.175	.298	.437	.053
N	12	12	12	12
Significance	.293	.173	.078	.435

[a]Massachusetts is omitted because 1970 data are missing.

Table A–12. Relationship Among Medically Needy Band, Utilization, and Expenditures, AFDC-Related Children, Twenty-eight States and District of Columbia with Medically Needy Programs, 1974

	1 Medically Needy Band 1974	2 Children under 21, 1974 (000)	3 Children Receiving Medical Services and No Cash Grant 1974 (000)	4 Children Recipients Divided by Child Pop. (3/2)	5 Expenditures for Medically Needy Children 1974 ($000)	6 Expenditures per Child Resident 1974 (5/2)	7 Expenditures per Child Recipient 1974 (5/3)
Arkansas	−$900	770	1	.001	427	$.55	$427.00
California	+936	7,631	236	.031	58,302	7.64	247.04
Connecticut	+16	1,114	23	.021	4,585	4.12	199.35
D.C.	+252	251	21	.084	7,201	28.69	342.90
Hawaii	−288	341	4	.012	1,175	3.45	293.75
Illinois	+144	4,174	38	.009	8,028	1.92	211.26
Kansas	+1,016	831	11	.013	6,222	7.49	565.64
Kentucky	+992	1,283	44	.034	4,239	3.30	96.34
Maine	−588	398	1	.003	172	.43	172.00
Maryland	+488	1,563	38	.024	7,693	4.92	202.45
Massachusetts	+1,652	2,105	93	.044	23,076	10.96	248.13
Michigan	+100	3,614	61	.017-	47,785	13.22	783.36
Minnesota	+60	1,527	25	.016	11,775	7.71	471.00
Montana	+1,262	287	—	—	—	—	—

Nebraska	−84	581	4	.007	367	.63	91.75
New Hampshire	+448	303	2	.007	234	.77	117.00
New York	−296	6,388	230	.036	151,322	23.69	657.92
North Carolina	+592	2,056	11	.005	2,166	1.05	196.91
North Dakota	−180	252	.6	.002	114	.45	190.00
Oklahoma	+868	986	21	.021	10,761	10.91	512.43
Pennsylvania	−188	4,192	96	.023	18,564	4.43	193.38
Rhode Island	+1,068	336	3	.009	553	1.65	184.33
Tennessee	−404	1,533	2	.001	330	.22	115.00
Utah	+112	526	6	.011	2,662	5.06	443.67
Vermont	−20	183	7	.038	2,039	11.14	291.29
Virginia	−262	1,870	18	.010	5,443	2.91	302.39
Washington	+468	1,295	44	.034	8,253	6.37	187.57
West Virginia	−404	648	7	.011	818	1.26	116.86
Wisconsin	+444	1,765	52	.029	28,439	16.06	546.90

Sources: Medically Needy Band from S. M. Davidson, "The Status of Aid to the Medically Needy," *Social Service Review*, March 1979, p. 96. Population of Children, U.S. Department of Commerce, *Statistical Abstract of the U.S., 1975*, table 36, p. 32. Medically Needy Recipients and Expenditures from *Numbers of Recipients and Amounts of Payments Under Medicaid, FY 1974*, table 7, p. 27, and table 18, p. 58 (USDHEW, Pub. No. (SRS) 77–03153.)

Table A-13. Relationship Among Medically Needy Band, Utilization, and Expenditures, Aged Couples in States with Medically Needy Programs, FY 1976

	1 Medically Needy Band FY 1976	2 Population Age 65 and Over 1976 (000)	3 Elderly Receiving Medical Services and No Cash Grant, 1976	4 Elderly Recipients Divided by Elderly Population (Col. 3/Col. 2)	5 Expenditures for Medically Needy Elderly 1976 ($000)	6 Expenditures per Elderly Resident 1976 (Col. 5/Col. 2)	7 Expenditures per Elderly Recipient (5/3)
States in Which Eligibility is Automatic with SSI							
Arkansas	-$935	277	13	0.047	$35,875	$129.51	2,759.62
California	-2,804	2,121	83	0.039	216,295	101.98	2,605.96
D.C.	-39	72	9	0.13	11,994	166.58	1,332.67
Kansas	+1,161	289	15	0.05	26,791	92.70	1,786.07
Kentucky	-639	373	13	0.03	22,527	60.39	1,732.85
Maine	-324	128	6	0.05	23,107	180.52	3,851.17
Maryland	-539	350	31	0.09	51,164	146.18	1,650.45
Massachusetts	-620	682	51	0.07	164,676	241.46	3,228.94
Michigan	+340	834	53	0.06	154,317	185.03	2,911.64
Montana	+261	77	4	0.05	10,609	137.78	2,652.25
New York	+356	2,068	172	0.08	1,089,369	526.77	6,333.54
North Dakota	-439	75	3	0.04	10,877	145.03	3,625.67

Pennsylvania	−704	1,404	110	0.08	205,528	146.39	1,868.44
Rhode Island	+448	116	24	0.21	32,258	278.09	1,344.08
Tennessee	−1,239	453	13	0.03	44,545	98.33	3,426.54
Vermont	−6	53	4	0.08	11,049	208.47	2,762.25
Washington	+144	374	23	0.06	36,178	96.73	1,572.96
West Virginia	−639	214					—
Wisconsin	+96	523	64	0.12	120,920	231.20	1,889.38
209(B) States							
Connecticut	−748	330	20	0.06	78,243	237.10	3,912.15
Hawaii	+220	60	5	0.08	14,442	240.70	2,888.40
Illinois	−439	1,171	74	0.06	144,163	123.11	1,948.15
Minnesota	0	445	36	0.08	120,907	271.70	3,358.53
Nebraska	−672	196	8	0.04	19,840	101.22	2,480.00
New Hampshire	+661	91	8	0.09	16,937	186.12	2,117.13
North Carolina	−1,739	513	20	0.04	37,910	73.90	1,895.50
Oklahoma	−492	339	6	0.02	14,818	43.71	2,469.67
Utah	−39	94	4	0.04	8,824	93.87	2,206.00
Virginia	−39	441	29	0.07	52,136	118.22	1,797.79

Table A-14.   Limitations on selected services offered under Title XIX

State	Inpatient Hospital Services	Skilled Nursing Facility Services	Intermediate Care Facility Services	Physicians' Services
Alabama	20 days per calendar year.	Preauthorization required.	Preauthorization required.	Prior authorization required, 1 visit per month outside hospital for chronic stable illness; 1 visit per day in hospital.
Alaska	Nonemergency out-of-state hospitalization requires preauthorization.	do	do	Elective (cosmetic) surgery requires preauthorization.
Arkansas	Limited to 25 days per calendar year with provision for extension based on medical necessity and with prior autorization.	No limitations. Prior authorization required.	No limitations.	18 visits per calendar year in physician's office, patient's home or nursing home. For hospital emergency room visits, 12 per calendar year.
California	Subject to prior authorization and specified length of stay as approved.	Subject to preadmission authorization and periodic reauthorization.	Subject to preadmission authorization and periodic reauthorization.	Except for services to inpatients of hospitals, nursing homes and intermediate care facilities, limited to a total of 2 occasions of service per month unless approval is obtained for an extended treatment plan. Services for cosmetic purposes not covered.
Colorado	Services provided as long as is medically necessary. Emergency hospital services provided when necessary to prevent death or serious impairment of health, even though hospital may not meet conditions for participation under Title XVIII.	No limitations.	No limitations.	12 home and office calls per calendar year.

State				
Connecticut	Prior authorization is required beyond 10 days.	Initial review to determine level of care made by a medical consultant within 14 days of patient's admission to a facility. Periodic patient reviews are made thereafter by a team to determine need for skilled nursing services.	Level of care is determined within 14 days of patient's admission to facility and the need for continued care in the facility is periodically determined thereafter.	Prior authorization required for services to patients in skilled nursing homes beyond 1 visit per month for chronic conditions and 5 visits per month for acute conditions.
Delaware	No limitations.	No limitations.	No limitations.	No limitations.
District of Columbia	Services provided in connection with surgical procedures for cosmetic purposes (except for emergency repair of accidental injury) will be included only by prior authorization issued by State agency; services provided in connection with dental or oral surgery will be limited to those required for emergency repair of accidental injury to jaw and related structures.	Items and services furnished by skilled nursing homes maintained primarily for care and treatment of inpatients with TB will be provided only for individuals 65 years of age or older.	do	Elective procedures requiring general anesthesia will be provided only when performed in a facility accredited for such procedures. Surgical procedures for cosmetic purposes (except for emergency repair of accidental injury) will be provided only by prior authorization issued by State agency. Ambulatory psychiatric care will be provided only in a formally organized psychiatric clinic which is approved as such by State agency, except when prior authorization for such care has been obtained from State agency.
Florida	45 days per patient per fiscal year.	No limitations.	No limitations.	No specified limitations.

Table A-14. Continued

State	Inpatient Hospital Services	Skilled Nursing Facility Services	Intermediate Care Facility Services	Physicians' Services
Georgia	Prior approval required for renal dialysis and/or kidney transplants except in cases of emergency dialysis which requires a notation on claim form that such treatment was an emergency.	Initial prior approval is required.	Initial prior approval is required.	Outpatient psychotherapy is limited to maximum of $250 per patient per calendar year. Unless medically justifiable need for exception exists, home and office visits limited to 1 per month, nursing home visits limited to 1 per month, and hospital visits limited to 1 per day.
Guam	Categorically needy—no limitations. Medically needy—Not more than 65 days at semiprivate rate. 1 doctor visit per day except for intensive care or consultation. 1st 3 pints of blood.	No limitations.	Not provided.	3 routine visits per month. Not to exceed 36 in 12 mo-period. 2 visits per week in SNF.
Hawaii	Hospital admissions are authorized for following number of days: Medical and surgical—8 days. Confinement and delivery—4 days. T. & A.—2 days. Psychiatric—10 days. Prior or authorization is required for any nonemergency admission such as for elective surgery: approval for extension is required for additional days.	Prior authorization required.	Prior authorization required.	For patients in skilled nursing facilities limited to 2 visits per month except during acute episodes when additional visits are authorized.

State				
Idaho	Limited to 20 days per admission. Abortion related services will not be provided unless the abortion or abortion related services are recommended by 2 consulting physicians who state that it is necessary to save the life or health of the mother, or unless the pregnancy is a result of rape or incest as determined by the courts.	Prior authorization is required before payment.	Prior authorization is required before payment.	Physician services related to abortion or abortion related services will not be provided unless the abortion or abortion related services are recommended by 2 consulting physicians who state that it is necessary to save the life or health of the mother, or unless the pregnancy is a result of rape or incest as determined by the courts.
Illinois	No limitations.	No limitations.	No limitations.	No limitations.
Indiana	do	do	do	Do.
Iowa	do	do	do	Do.
Kansas	do	do	do	Do.
Kentucky	21 days per admission.	Preauthorization required.	Preauthorization required.	Initial and extensive visits limited to 2 per calendar year. Preauthorization required for those patients who are "locked in" to 1 physician visit and 1 pharmacy, who require services in excess of 4 prescriptions and 4 physician office visits per month.
Louisiana	No limitations.	No limitations.	No limitations.	Limited to 12 visits per year, with extensions subject to prior approval.
Maine	No limitations—Prior authorization required for private duty nursing, intensive care services, private room, and extension of hospital benefits days beyond 60 days.	No limitations. Prior authorization required for private duty nursing and private room.	do	Do.

Table A-14.   Continued

State	Inpatient Hospital Services	Skilled Nursing Facility Services	Intermediate Care Facility Services	Physicians' Services
Maryland	Preauthorization required.	Preauthorization required for all admissions.	Preauthorization required for all admissions.	Preauthorization required for surgery normally considered cosmetic.
Massachusetts	No Limitations.	No Limitations.	No limitations	Routine visits to patients shall be limited to 1 visit per month, unless medical justification is submitted to verify need for additional visits. Multiple monthly visits on chronic basis require written approval from regional medical unit.
Michigan	Minimum period necessary in type of facility for the proper care and treatment of patient.	Minimum period necessary in type of facility for the proper care and treatment of patient.	Provided based on level of care appropriate to patient's medical needs.	No specified limitations.
Minnesota	No limitations.	No limitations.	No limitations.	No limitations.
Mississippi	40 days per fiscal year.	Prior authorization required.	Prior authorization required.	Hospital visits—limited to 1 per day; nursing home visits—limited to 36 per fiscal year.
Missouri	21 days per admission.	do	Not provided.	Limited to those that are medically necessary. Payment is not made for cosmetic surgery. Certain recipients who have over-utilized physician's services are limited to service of only 1 physician of their own choosing.
Montana	30 days per fiscal year.	No limitations.	No limitations.	No limitations.
Nebraska	Acute inpatient psychiatric care—14 days with extension.	do	do	No specified limitations.

State				
Nevada	No limitations.	do	do	No limitations.
New Hampshire	Requires prior approval for patients who are anticipated to require hospitalization for period longer than 12 days.	Prior authorization required.	Prior authorization required.	1 physician visit per month in ICF; 1 physician visit per week in SNF.
New Jersey	Limited by exclusion of elective surgery and diet therapy for exogenous obesity.	Prior authorization required except where patient is transferred to nursing home directly from an acute care facility.	do	Prior authorization required for elective cosmetic surgery and for psychiatric treatment when costs exceed $300 in given year.
New Mexico	No limitations.	No limitations.	No limitations.	No limitations.
New York	No limitations. (Revisions under consideration.)	Prior approval except when admitted directly from hospital, another nursing home, or from health related facility.	do	Do.
North Carolina	Prior authorization required for admissions for cosmetic surgery and surgical transplants except bone and tendon transplants.	Prior approval required.	Prior authorization required.	Routine physical exams and routine screening tests are excluded except for EPSDT recipients and an annual examination allowed for recipients in homes for aged, skilled nursing homes, and intermediate care facilities. Eye refractions are limited to 1 per year for recipients ages 24 and under, and 1 in 2 years for recipients ages 25 and over. Prior approval required for surgical transplants (except for bone and tendon), cosmetic surgery and more than 2 psychiatric visits.
North Dakota	No limitations.	No limitations.	No limitations.	No limitations.

Table A-14. Continued

State	Inpatient Hospital Services	Skilled Nursing Facility Services	Intermediate Care Facility Services	Physicians' Services
Ohio	90-day limitation per spell of illness.	Physicians' certification and recertification required every 50 days.	No limitations. Person must be in need of such care.	10 physician visits per month.
Oklahoma	10 days per admission.	No limitation.	Preauthorization required.	Categorically needy: Inpatient hospital visits—limited for compensable hospital periods; outpatient—4 office visits per month: 2 visits per month in nursing home. Medically needy: Inpatient limited to hospital visits and surgical services for a compensable period of hospitalization; outpatient—4 home visits per month; nursing homes—2 visits per month.
Oregon	Limited to 21 days.	No limitations.	No limitations.	Prior authorization required for elective and rehabilitative procedures.
Pennsylvania	60 days of intermittent or consecutive care in a benefit period.	do	do	Prior authorization required for all general and special medical examinations and consultations. Hospital inpatients—consultations limited to 1 per specialty per hospital admission; outpatient—consultation limited to 1 per 12 mo. period. $200 maximum amount during any 1 period of hospitalization or for a series of recurrent or related surgical procedures.

State				
Puerto Rico	Limited to services provided in public facilities and some private facilities under contract.	Provided in eligible public facilities and in some private facilities under contract.	Not provided.	Available in public facilities and through some physicians under contract.
Rhode Island	Prior authorization required for stays in excess of 15 days per admission for persons under age 65, or in excess of 60 days for persons age 65 or older who are also covered by medicare.	Prior authorization required for all admissions.	Prior authorization required.	Prior authorization required for visits in excess of 2 per month for chronic illness and in excess of 8 per month for acute illness; inpatient hospital visits in excess of 37 days up to maximum of 100 days, office visits provided by psychiatrists beyond initial evaluation visit.
South Carolina	40 days per fiscal year.	Need for care approved or disapproved by State office.	Need for care approved or disapproved by State office.	Must be medically justified.
South Dakota	30 days per benefit period, 1st 3 pints of blood per benefit period.	No limitations.	No limitations.	Limitations to services which are medically necessary and required by patient.
Tennessee	20 days per fiscal year.	Prior authorization required.	do	Prior approval required for unusual elective types of surgical procedures.
Texas	30 days per spell of illness.	Level of care determination is required.	Level of care determination is required.	No limitations.
Utah	60 days per spell of illness.	No limitations.	No limitations.	No limitations on number of visits for acute conditions, except psychiatric care is limited to 12 hours of treatment for each acute illness unless prior written approval for additional care is obtained.
Vermont	No specified day limitations.	Authorization is required.	Authorization is required.	Treatment of mental, psychoneurotic or personality disorders limited to $500 per calendar year.

Table A–14.   Continued

State	Inpatient Hospital Services	Skilled Nursing Facility Services	Intermediate Care Facility Services	Physicians' Services
Virgin Islands	No specified limitations	Service presently being developed. Prior authorization will be required.	Not provided.	No specified limitations.
Virginia	14 days per admission.	No limitations.	No limitations.	No limitations.
Washington	Approval for admission required.	Prior approval of admission.	do	1 visit per month in office, home, skilled nursing facility, intermediate care facility for nonemergency conditions. 2 per month in extended care facility. 2 calls for new and acute conditions. 1 per day in hospital, additional calls must be justified.
West Virginia	No limitations.	No limitations.	do	No limitations.
Wisconsin	do	No limitations; prior authorization required.	No limitations; prior authorization required.	Do.
Wyoming	14 days per spell of illness.	No limitations.	No limitations.	Physical examinations limited to 1 yearly after 3rd year of life; nursing home visits limited to 1 routine visit per month.

Source: Health Care Financing Administration, Medicaid Bureau, *Data on the Medicaid Program: Eligibility, Services, Expenditures, Fiscal Years 1966–1977.* Washington, D.C.: U.S. Department of Health, Education, and Welfare, 1977, pp. 7–11.

Table A–15.   The Use of Limitations and Prior Authorization by States for Seven Mandatory Medicaid Services, June 1975.

State	Inpatient Hospital Services	Outpatient Hospital Services	Laboratory and X-ray	Skilled Nursing	Physicians' Services	EPSDT	Family Planning
Alabama	1	2	2	1	1	1	2
Alaska	2	2	2	1	2	1	2
Arizona	—	—	—	—	—	—	—
Arkansas	1	1	1	2	1	2	1
California	1	1	2	1	1	2	2
Colorado	2	2	2	2	1	1	2
Connecticut	1	1	2	1	1	1	2
Delaware	2	2	2	2	2	2	2
D.C.	2	1	1	2	1	2	2
Florida	1	1	1	1	1	1	1
Georgia	2	2	2	2	1	2	2
Guam	2	2	2	2	2	2	2
Hawaii	0	0	1	1	1	1	2
Idaho	1	2	2	2	2	2	2
Illinois	2	2	2	2	2	1	2
Indiana	2	2	2	2	2	1	2
Iowa	2	2	2	1	1	1	2
Kansas	1	2	2	2	1	1	2
Kentucky	0	1	2	2	2	2	2
Louisiana	1	1	2	2	2	2	2
Maine	1	1	2	2	2	1	2
Maryland	1	1	2	1	1	1	2
Massachusetts	2	2	2	2	1	1	2
Michigan	2	2	2	2	2	2	2
Minnesota	2	2	2	2	2	2	2
Mississippi	1	1	2	1	1	1	2
Missouri	1	1	1	1	1	1	2
Montana	1	1	1	2	2	1	2
Nebraska	1	2	2	2	1	2	2
Nevada	0	2	2	0	1	2	2
New Hampshire	0	2	2	0	1	1	2
New Jersey	1	1	2	1	1	1	2
New Mexico	1	2	2	2	1	1	2
New York	1	2	2	1	2	2	2
North Carolina	2	1	2	1	2	2	2
North Dakota	2	2	2	2	2	2	2
Ohio	2	2	2	2	1	2	2
Oklahoma	1	1	1	1	1	1	2
Oregon	1	2	2	2	1	2	2
Pennsylvania	1	1	1	2	2	1	2
Puerto Rico	2	2	2	2	2	1	2
Rhode Island	0	1	2	1	0	2	2
South Carolina	1	2	2	1	2	1	2
South Dakota	1	2	2	2	1	1	2
Tennessee	1	1	1	0	1	1	2
Texas	1	2	2	2	1	1	2
Utah	1	2	2	2	1	1	2
Vermont	2	2	2	0	1	1	2
Virgin Islands	2	2	2	1	2	2	2
Virginia	1	2	2	2	1	2	2
Washington	0	1	1	1	1	1	2
West Virginia	1	2	2	0	2	2	2
Wisconsin	2	2	2	2	2	2	2
Wyoming	1	2	2	2	1	1	2
Summary:	0= 6	0= 1	0= 0	0= 5	0= 2	0= 0	0= 0
	1=28	1=19	1=10	1=18	1=30	1=30	1= 2
	2=19	2=33	2=43	2=30	2=21	2=23	2=51

Source: Commerce Clearing House, *Medicare and Medicaid Guide,* State Plans.

Key: 0 = limits and prior authorization; 1 = limits and no prior authorization, or prior authorization and no limits; 2 = no limits and no prior authorization.

Table A–16.   Changes in Optional Services and Limitations on Five Basic Services, by State, 1970–1975

	Optional Services[a]			Limitations[b]		
	1970	1975	Change	1970	1975	Change
Alabama	2	2		3	3	
Alaska	no prog	2		no prog	4	
Arizona	no prog			no prog.		
Arkansas	2	3	+1	1	3	+2
California	3	4	+1	3	3	
Colorado	2	2		2	4	+2
Connecticut	3	4	+1	4	3	−1
Delaware	2	2		4	4	
D.C.	2	3	+1	3	4	+1
Florida	3	2	−1	0	3	+1
Georgia	2	3	+1	4	4	
Hawaii	3	3		3	2	−1
Idaho	2	2		3	4	+1
Illinois	3	4	+1	4	4	
Indiana	4	3	−1	4	4	
Iowa	3	4	+1	3	4	+1
Kansas	3	4	+1	3	4	+1
Kentucky	2	3	+1	3	2	−1
Louisiana	2	3	+1	2	3	+1
Maine	3	4	+1	4	4	
Maryland	3	3		3	3	
Massachusetts	3	4	+1	4	4	
Michigan	2	4	+2	2	4	+2
Minnesota	3	4	+1	2	4	+2
Mississippi	2	2		2	3	+1
Missouri	3	2	−1	3	3	
Montana	3	4	+1	3	3	
Nebraska	3	4	+1	3	4	+1
Nevada	3	4	+1	2	3	+1
New Hampshire	4	3	−1	2	3	+1
New Jersey	3	4	+1	3	3	
New Mexico	3	3		3	4	+1
New York	3	4	+1	4	4	
North Carolina	3	3		2	4	+2
North Dakota	3	4	+1	2	4	+2
Ohio	3	4	+1	2	4	+2
Oklahoma	2	2		2	3	+1
Oregon	3	4	+1	3	4	+1
Pennsylvania	2	3	+1	2	3	+1
Rhode Island	2	2		2	3	+1
South Carolina	3	4	+1	3	4	+1
South Dakota	2	3	+1	4	4	
Tennessee	3	2	−1	3	3	
Texas	2	3	+1	2	4	+2
Utah	3	4	+1	3	4	+1
Vermont	3	3	+1	3	3	
Virginia	3	3		3	4	+1
Washington	3	4	+1	2	3	+1
West Virginia	3	4	+1	2	4	+2
Wisconsin	4	4		3	4	+1
Wyoming	1	1		2	4	+2

Source: S. M. Davidson, "Variations in State Medicaid Programs," J. of Health Politics, Policy, and Law, Spring 1978, pp. 56–57, 60–61.

[a]Optional services	Number provided	0	Coded score:	0
		1–4		1
		5–9		2
		10–14		3
		15–		4

[b]Limitations on provision of services for
each basic service if there are:
Limits and prior authorization required =0
Limits but no limits prior authorization required
or no limits but prior authorization
is required   =1
no limits and no prior authorization   =2
if the total score for all 5 basic services

combined is:	0	Then codes are:	0
	1–2		1
	3–5		2
	6–8		3
	9–10		4

Table A-17.   Population, Recipients, and Expenditures, Thirteen States, 1975

	State Population (000)	Medicaid Recipients	Medicaid Expenditures ($)	Medicaid Expenditures per State Resident ($)	Medicaid Expenditures per Recipient ($)
Indiana	5,311	242,184	172,434	32.47	712.00
Iowa	2,870	143,335	81,699	28.47	569.99
Nebraska	1,546	69,624	54,269	35.10	779.46
Texas	12,237	728,698	460,632	37.64	632.13
California	21,185	3,344,341	1,491,088	70.38	445.85
Massachusetts	5,828	589,848	493,695	84.71	836.99
New York	18,120	2,974,330	2,954,622	163.06	993.37
Georgia	4,926	516,325	256,270	52.02	496.33
Oklahoma	2,712	216,978	140,647	51.86	648.21
Tennessee	4,188	319,600	122,701	29.30	383.92
Colorado	2,534	151,415	98,030	38.69	693.21
Maryland	4,098	399,128	187,300	45.71	469.27
Pennsylvania	11,827	1,331,230	709,150	59.96	532.70

Sources: State Population: U.S. Bureau of the Census, *Statistical Abstract of the U.S., 1976* (Washington, D.C.: USGPO, 1976), Table 10, p. 11. Medicaid Recipients and Expenditures: OPPR/HCFA/USDHEW, *Medicaid State Tables, FY 1975* (Washington, D.C.: USGPO, 1978), Tables 2, 3, pp. 7–10.

Table A–18. Population, Users of Services under Medicaid, Total Medicaid Expenditures, and Expenditures on Physician Services under Medicaid, by State, 1975

State	State Population (thousands)	Users of Services under Medicaid (thousands)	Total Medicaid Expenditures (thousands of dollars)	Medicaid Expenditures on Physician Services (thousands of dollars)
Alabama	3614	323	131336	16415
Alaska	352	10	8515	1307
Arkansas	2116	184	93005	8796
California	21185	3344	1491088	234443
Colorado	2534	151	98030	9771
Connecticut	3095	192	161075	11973
Delaware	579	49	14626	2622
D. C.	716	147	94101	13893
Florida	8357	386	172676	18771
Georgia	4926	516	256270	36528
Hawaii	865	109	36953	5684
Idaho	820	39	24460	3326
Illinois	11145	1600	682409	94021
Indiana	5311	242	172434	13714
Iowa	2870	143	81699	8532
Kansas	2267	155	101947	10597
Kentucky	3396	357	100280	12860
Louisiana	3791	397	143309	10696
Maine	1059	122	60407	9948
Maryland	4098	399	187300	17554
Massachusetts	5828	590	493695	33033
Michigan	9157	955	623251	90465
Minnesota	3926	245	255132	18111
Mississippi	2346	287	93742	15425
Missouri	4763	360	99284	16616
Montana	748	45	29096	4342
Nebraska	1546	70	54269	4392
Nevada	592	23	16149	2383
New Hampshire	818	50	28185	3800
New Jersey	7316	623	366407	43715
New Mexico	1147	76	28961	4258
New York	18120	2974	2954622	148011
North Carolina	5451	329	163231	19519
North Dakota	635	27	23463	1823
Ohio	10759	764	366292	44694
Oklahoma	2712	217	149647	15902
Oregon	2288	169	74141	5293
Pennsylvania	11827	1331	709150	42994
Rhode Island	927	109	72079	4538
South Carolina	2818	266	75692	9942
South Dakota	683	42	21759	2124
Tennessee	4188	320	122701	15525
Texas	12237	729	460632	53501
Utah	1206	56	30583	3341
Vermont	471	49	31282	4051
Virginia	4967	312	159625	19548
Washington	3544	288	176065	21334
West Virginia	1803	125	28919	5538
Wisconsin	4607	419	361237	23607
Wyoming	374	11	4887	745

Sources: Column 1: U.S. Bureau of the Census, *Statistical Abstract of the United States, 1976:28;* Columns 2–4: Health Care Financing Administration, *State Tables Fiscal Year 1975: Medicaid: Recipients, Payments, and Services,* 1978: Tables 1 and 5.

Bibliography

Aday, L. A. 1976. "The Impact of Health Policy on Access to Medical Care." *Milbank Memorial Fund Quarterly* 54:215—233.

Aday, L., and R. Eichhorn. 1973. *Utilization of Health Services Indices and Correlates: A Research Bibliography.* Washington, D.C.: U.S. Department of Health, Education and Welfare, Pub. No. (HSM) 73-3003.

American Medical Association. 1978. *Profile of Medical Practice.* Chicago: Center for Health Services Research and Development, American Medical Association.

Andersen, R.; J. Kravits; and O. W. Anderson, eds. 1975. *Equity in Health Services: Empirical Analyses in Social Policy.* Cambridge: Ballinger Publishing Company.

Andersen, R; J. Lion; and O. W. Anderson. 1976. *Two Decades of Health Services: Social Survey Trends in Use and Expenditure.* Cambridge: Ballinger Publishing Company.

Andersen, R., and J. F. Newman. 1973. "Societal and Individual Determinants of Medical Care Utilization in the United States." *Milbank Memorial Fund Quarterly* 51:95—124.

Anderson, O. W. 1968. *The Uneasy Equilibrium.* New Haven: College and University Press.

Bice, T. W.; R. L. Eichhorn; and P. D. Fox. 1972. "Socioeconomic Status and Use of Physician Services: A Reconsideration." *Medical Care* 10:261—271.

Blalock, Jr., H. M. 1972. *Social Statistics.* 2nd Edition. New York: McGraw-Hill Book Company.

Blanken, A. J. 1976. *Hospital Discharges and Length of Stay.* Vital and Health Statistics, Series 10, no. 107. DHEW Pub. No. (HRA)

77—1534. Rockville, Maryland: U.S. Public Health Service, Health Resources Administration.

Blim, R. D.; J. E. Strain; J. P. Connelly; and H. D. Taylor. 1979. "Pediatrics as a Primary, Secondary, and Tertiary Care Specialty: Cost and Reimbursement Implications." *Pediatrics* 63:659—661.

Boulding, K. 1973. "The Concept of Need for Health Services." In *Aspects of Health Care,* edited by J. B. McKinley. New York: Milbank Memorial Fund.

Bucher, B. M.; P. M. Gertman; and D. L. Rabin. 1972. "Inappropriate Patient Hospital Days Related to Patient, Disease, Physician, and Hospital Characteristics." Paper presented at the 53rd Annual Session of the American College of Physicians, Altantic City, New Jersey, April 30.

Bunker, J. 1970. "Surgical Manpower: A Comparison of Operations and Surgeons in the United States, in England, and Wales." *New England Journal of Medicine* 282:135—144.

Burney, I. L.; G. J. Schieber; M. O. Blaxall; and J. R. Gabel. 1978. "Geographic Variation in Physicians' Fees: Payments to Physicians Under Medicare and Medicaid." *Journal of the American Medical Association* 240:1368—1371.

Children's Defense Fund. 1977. *EPSDT: Does It Spell Health Care for Poor Children?* Washington, D.C.: Children's Defense Fund.

Commerce Clearing House. 1979. *Medicare and Medicaid Reporter.* Chicago: Commerce Clearing House.

Congressional Budget Office. 1979. *The Effect of PSROs on Health Care Costs: Current Findings and Future Evaluations.* Washington, D.C.: U.S. Government Printing Office.

Connecticut General Assembly, Legislative Program Review and Investigations Committee. 1976. *Containing Medicaid Costs in Connecticut.* Hartford, Connecticut, September.

Cooper, B. S.; N. L. Worthington; and M. F. McGee. 1976. *Compendium of National Health Expenditures Data.* DHEW Pub. No. (SSA) 76—11927. Washington, D.C.: U.S. Government Printing Office.

Davidson, S. M. Forthcoming. "Medicaid: The Issue of Physician Participation." In *Social Work and Health Care Policy,* edited by D. Lum. New York: Haworth Press.

———. 1979. "The Status of Aid to the Medically Needy." *Social Service Review* (March):92—105.

———. 1978a. "Understanding the Growth of Emergency Department Utilization." *Medical Care* 16:122—132.

———. 1978b. "Variations in State Medicaid Programs." *Journal of Health Politics, Policy and Law* 3:54—70.

———. 1977. "Mode of Payment and Length of Stay in the Hospital: More Work for PSROs?" *Medical Care* 15:515—525.

———. 1974. *Report to the Medicaid Investigations Committee.* Springfield, Illinois: Illinois Department of Public Aid.

Davidson, S. M., and T. R. Marmor, with J. D. Perloff; N. Aitken; and M. Spear. 1980. *The Cost of Living Longer: National Health Insurance and the Elderly.* Lexington, Massachusetts: Lexington Books.

Davis, K., and R. Reynolds. 1976. "The Impact of Medicare and Medicaid on Access to Medical Care." In *The Role of Health Insurance in the Health Services Sector,* edited by R. N. Rosett. Neale Watson Academic Publications for National Bureau of Economic Research.

Davis, K., and C. Schoen. 1978. *Health and the War on Poverty: A Ten-Year Appraisal.* Washington, D.C.: The Brookings Institution.

Enthoven, A. C. 1978a. "Consumer-Choice Plan (First of Two Parts). Inflation and Inequity in Health Care Today: Alternatives for Cost Control and an Analysis of Proposals for National Health Insurance." *New England Journal of Medicine* 298:650—658.

———. 1978b. "Consumer-Choice Health Plan (Second of Two Parts). A National-Health-Insurance Proposal Based on Regulated Competition in the Private Sector." *New England Journal of Medicine* 298:709—720.

———. 1978c. "Shattuck Lecture—Cutting Cost Without Cutting the Quality of Care." *New England Journal of Medicine* 298:1229—1238.

Evans, R. 1974. "Supplier-Induced Demand: Some Empirical Evidence and Implications." *The Economics of Health and Medical Care,* edited by M. Perlman. New York: John Wiley and Sons.

Feldstein, M. S. 1971. *Rising Cost of Hospital Care.* Washington, D.C.: Information Resources Press.

Foltz, A. M., and D. Brown. 1975. "State Response to Federal Policy: Children, EPSDT, and the Medicaid Muddle." *Medical Care* 13:630—642.

Foster, R. W. 1977. "HMOs: A Synthesis of the Evidence of Use." Unpublished paper, University of Chicago Center for Health Administration Studies, April.

Gabel, J. R., and M. A. Redisch. 1979. "Alternative Physician Payment Methods: Incentives, Efficiency, and National Health Insurance." *Milbank Memorial Fund Quarterly* 57:38—59.

Garner, D. D.; W. C. Liao; and T. R. Sharpe. 1979. "Factors Affecting Physician Participation in a State Medicaid Program." *Medical Care* 17:43—58.

Gibson, R. M., and M. S. Mueller. 1977. "National Health Expenditures, Fiscal Year 1976." *Social Security Bulletin* 40:3—22.

Gibson, R. M., and C. R. Fisher. 1978. "National Health Expenditures, Fiscal Year 1977." *Social Security Bulletin* 41:3—20.

Harvard Child Health Project Task Force. 1977. *Vol. 1.: Toward a Primary Medical Care System Responsive to Children's Needs.* Cambridge: Ballinger Publishing Company.

Health Care Financing Administration, Medicaid Bureau. 1978. *Data on the Medicaid Program: Eligibility, Services, Expenditures Fiscal Years 1966—1978.* Washington, D.C.: U.S. Government Printing Office.

Hershey, J. C.; H. S. Luft; and J. M. Gianaris. 1975. "Making Sense Out of Utilization Data." *Medical Care* 13:838—854.

Holahan, J. *Financing Health Care for the Poor.* 1975. Lexington, Mass.: Lexington Books.

Holahan, J.; B. Spitz; W. Pollak; and J. Feder. 1977. *Altering Medicaid Provider Reimbursement Methods.* Washington, D.C.: The Urban Institute.

Hughes, Edward F. X. 1975. Statement presented to the Subcommittee on Oversight and Investigations of the House Committee on Interstate and Foreign Commerce, July 18, 1975. Washington, D.C.: U.S. Government Printing Office.

Illinois Economic and Fiscal Commission. 1976. *Medicaid Costs and Controls: An Analysis.* Springfield, Illinois: Illinois Economic and Fiscal Commission.

Keniston, K., and The Carnegie Council on Children. 1977. *All Our Children.* New York: Harcourt Brace Jovanovich.

Kravits, J., and J. Schneider. 1975. "Health Care Need and Actual Use by Age, Race and Income." In *Equity in Health Services: Empirical Analyses in Social Policy,* edited by R. Andersen, J. Kravits, and O. W. Anderson. Cambridge: Ballinger Publishing Company.

Kushman, J. E. 1977. "Physician Participation in Medicaid." *Western Journal of Agricultural Economics* 2:21—33.

Marmor, T. R. 1973. *The Politics of Medicare.* Chicago: Aldine.

Marmor, T. R.; W. L. Hoffman; and T. C. Heagy. 1975. "National Health Insurance: Some Lessons from the Canadian Experience." *Policy Sciences* 6:447—466.

Massachusetts Medical Society. 1979. *Newsletter.* (January).

McCarthy, E. G., and G. Widmer. 1974. "Effects of Screening by Consultants on Recommended Elective Surgical Procedures." *New England Journal of Medicine* 291:1331 —1335.

Mesel, E., and D. D. Wirtschafter. 1976. "Automation of a Patient Medical Profile from Insurance Claims Data: A Possible First Step in Automating Ambulatory Medical Records on a National Scale." *Milbank Memorial Fund Quarterly* 54:29—45.

Monsma, G. 1970. "Marginal Revenue and the Demand for Physicians' Services." In *Empirical Studies in Health Economics,* edited by H. Klarman. Baltimore: Johns Hopkins University Press.

Moore, S. 1979. "Cost Containment Through Risk-Sharing by Primary Care Physicians." *New England Journal of Medicine* 300 (1979): 1359—1362.

National Center for Health Statistics. 1975. *Physician Visits, Volume and Interval Since Last Visit: United States—1971.* Vital and Health Statistics, Series 10, No. 97, DHEW Pub. No. (HRA) 75—1524. Rockville, Maryland: U.S. Department of Health, Education and Welfare, Health Resources Administration.

———. 1966. *Hospital Discharges and Length of Stay: Short-Stay Hospitals. United States—July 1963—June 1964.* Vital and Health Statistics, Series 10, No. 30, DHEW Pub. No. (PHS) 1000. Washington, D.C.: U.S. Department of Health, Education and Welfare, Public Health Service.

———. 1965a. *Volume of Physician Visits by Place of Visit and Type of Service.* United States—July 1963—June 1964. Vital and Health Statistics, Series 10, No. 18, DHEW Pub. No. (PHS) 1000. Washington, D.C.: U.S. Department of Health, Education and Welfare. Public Health Service.

———. 1965b. *Physician Visits. Interval of Visits and Children's Routine Checkup.* United States—July 1963—June 1964. Vital and Health Statistics, Series 10, No. 19, DHEW Pub. No. (PHS) 1000. Washington, D.C.: U.S. Department of Health, Education and Welfare, Public Health Service.

———. 1964. *Medical Care, Health Status and Family Income. United States.* Vital and Health Statistics, Series 10, No. 9, DHEW pub. No. (PHS) 1000. Washington, D.C.: U.S. Department of Health, Education and Welfare, Public Health Service.

National Center for Social Statistics. 1974. *Medicaid Recipient Characteristics and Units of Selected Medical Services, 1972. NCSS Report B—4 Supplement.* Washington, D.C.: U.S. Government Printing Office.

———. 1972. *Medicaid and Other Medical Care Financed from Public Assistance Funds. Fiscal Year 1971. NCSS Report B—5.* Washington, D.C.: U.S. Government Printing Office.

———. 1970, 1972, 1974, 1976. *Public Assistance Statistics NCSS Report A—2.* Washington, D.C.: U.S. Government Printing Office. February 1970, August 1970, February 1972, August 1972, February 1974, August 1974, February 1976, August 1976.

———. 1968, 1970, 1972, 1974, 1976. *Medical Assistance (Medicaid) Financed Under Title XIX of the Social Security Act. NCSS Report B —1.* Washington, D.C.: U.S. Government Printing Office, February 1968, August 1968, February 1970, August 1970, February 1972, August 1972, February 1974, August 1974, February 1976, August 1976.

————. 1968, 1969, 1970, 1972, 1973, 1974. *Numbers of Recipients and Amounts of Payments Under Medicaid. NCSS Report B—4.* Washington, D.C: U.S. Government Printing Office.

National Governor's Conference Task Force. 1977. *Report on Medicaid Reform.* Washington, D.C.: U.S. Government Printing Office.

Okun, A. M. *Equality and Efficiency: The Big Tradeoff.* 1975. Washington, D.C.: The Brookings Institution.

Physician's Management Staff. 1978. "Is Anybody Happy with Medicaid?" *Physician's Management* (November) 34—37.

Roemer, M. I. 1961. "Bed Supply and Hospital Utilization: A Natural Experiment." *Hospitals* 35:36—42.

Rosenberg, S. N.; C. Gunston; L. Berenson; and A. Klein. 1976. "An Eclectic Approach to Quality Control in Fee-for-Service Health Care: The New York City Medicaid Experience." *American Journal of Public Health* 66:21—30.

Schieber, G. J.; I. L. Burney; J. Golden; and W. A. Kraus. 1976. "Physician Fee Patterns Under Medicare: A Descriptive Analysis." *New England Journal of Medicine* 294:1089—1093.

Schultze, C. L. 1977. *The Public Use of Private Interest.* Washington, D.C.: The Brookings Institution.

Sloan, F.; J. Cromwell; and J. B. Mitchell. 1977. *A Study of Administrative Costs in Physicians' Offices and Medicaid Participation, Final Report.* Cambridge: Abt Associates, Inc.

Somers, H. M., and A. R. Somers. 1967. *Medicare and the Hospitals: Issues and Prospects.* Washington, D.C.: The Brookings Institution.

Stevens, R. 1971. "Trends in Medical Specialization in the United States." *Inquiry* 8:9—19.

Stevens, R., and R. Stevens. 1974. *Welfare Medicine in America: A Case Study of Medicaid.* New York: Free Press.

Stuart, B. 1977. "Utilization Controls." In *Controlling Medical Utilization Patterns*, edited by J. Holahan and B. Stuart. Washington, D.C.: The Urban Institute.

"Supplemental Security Income for the Aged, Blind, and Disabled: Number of Persons Receiving Federally Administered Payments and Total Amount, By Reason of Eligibility, February and March 1974." 1974. *Social Security Bulletin* 37:56.

"Supplemental Security Income for the Aged, Blind, and Disabled: Number of Persons Receiving Federally Administered Payments and Total Amount, By Reason of Eligibility, August, 1974." 1974. *Social Security Bulletin* 37:65.

"Supplemental Security Income for the Aged, Blind, and Disabled: Number of Persons Receiving Federally Administered Payments and Total Amount, By Reason of Eligibility, August 1976." 1976. *Social Security Bulletin* 39:56.

Thorndike, N. 1977. "1975 Net Income and Work Patterns of Physicians in Five Medical Specialities." Research and Statistics Note

No. 13. HEW Pub. No. (SSA) 77-11701. Washington, D.C.: U.S. Government Printing Office.

Titmuss, R. M. 1968. "The Role of Redistribution in Social Policy." In *Commitment to Welfare,* edited by R. M. Titmuss. New York: Pantheon Books.

U.S. Bureau of Family Services. 1968. *Advance Release of Statistics on Public Assistance.* Washington, D.C.: U.S. Government Printing Office, February and August.

U.S. Bureau of the Census. 1976. *Historical Statistics of the United States, Part I.* Washington, D.C: U.S. Printing Office.

————. 1967, 1969, 1971, 1973, 1974, 1975. *Statistical Abstract of the United States.* Washington, D.C.: U.S. Government Printing Office.

U.S. Department of Health, Education and Welfare (HCFA). 1979. *Medicaid State Tables Fiscal Year 1978. Recipients, Payments and Services.* Washington, D.C.: U.S. Government Printing Office.

————. 1978a. *State Tables Fiscal Year 1975. Medicaid: Recipients, Payments and Services.* Washington, D.C.: U.S. Government Printing Office.

————. 1978b. *Medicaid State Tables Fiscal Year 1976. Recipients, Payments and Services.* Washington, D.C.: U.S. Government Printing Office.

U.S. Social Security Administration. 1974, 1976. *Social Security Bulletin.* Washington, D.C.: U.S. Government Printing Office, July 1974, December 1974, December 1976.

Vayda, E. 1973. "A Comparison of Surgical Rates in Canada and in England and Wales." *New England Journal of Medicine* 289:1224—1229.

Wennberg, J. 1975. Statement presented to the Subcommittee on Oversight and Investigations of the House Committee on Interstate and Foreign Commerce, July 15, 1975. Washington, D.C.: U.S. Government Printing Office.

Wennberg, J., and A. Gittelsohn. 1973. "Small Area Variations in Health Care Delivery." *Science* 182:1102—1108.

Wilensky, H. L., and C. N. Lebeaux. 1976. "Conceptions of Social Welfare." In *The Emergence of Social Welfare and Social Work,* edited by N. Gilbert and H. Specht. Itasca, Illinois: F. E. Peacock Publishers, Inc.

————. 1958. *Industrial Society and Social Welfare.* New York: Russell Sage Foundation.

Wolins, M. 1976. "The Societal Function of Social Welfare." In *The Emergence of Social Welfare and Social Work,* edited by N. Gilbert and H. Specht. Itasca, Illinois: F. E. Peacock Publishers, Inc.

Zimmer, J. G. 1974. "Length of Stay and Hospital Bed Misutilization." *Medical Care* 12:453—462.

Index

About the Author

Stephen M. Davidson has been on the faculty of the University of Chicago's School of Social Service Administration since 1971. He specializes in public policy relating to health and medical care in organizational planning. In addition to articles on Medicaid, Mr. Davidson is the author of papers on a variety of subjects including the utilization of emergency services, planning for ambulatory care, cost-sharing, and the use of non-physician personnel. He is currently pursuing some of the questions raised in this book in a HCFA-funded, thirteen-state study of physician participation in Medicaid. Mr. Davidson is also the co-author of a recent book, *The Cost of Living Longer: National Health Insurance and the Elderly,* and a monograph, *Effective Social Services for Older Americans.* He is a graduate of Swarthmore College, the University of Maryland, and the University of Chicago.